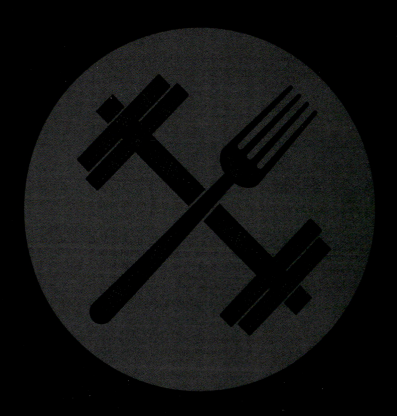

CLEAN SIMPLE EATS

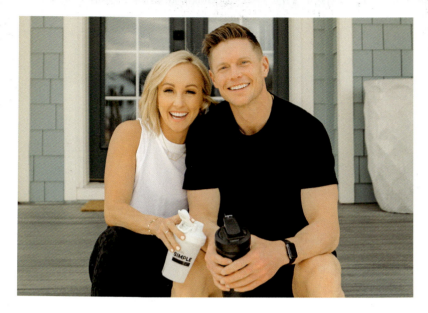

Every recipe book tells a story and this one begins with PROTEIN. This book is jam-packed with 100+ limited-edition recipes, each powered by our deliciously rich and creamy protein powder—all 17 flavors included. But there's more to this protein than meets the eye… we'll have you shaking, baking, and rolling from sun up to sun down, that's no lie!

Our classic flavors like Simply Vanilla, Brownie Batter, Caramel Toffee, and Chocolate PB are easy to love. You'll go bananas for our fruity flaves featuring Bananas Foster, Coconut Cream, Peaches & Cream, Strawberry Cheesecake, and Key Lime. When you're looking to spice it up, try our Pumpkin Pie, Eggnog, Snickerdoodle or Cinnamon Roll—made with (no sugar) spice and everything nice. For a special treat, indulge in our Mint Chocolate Cookie, Maple Donut, Cake Batter or S'mores! Spoiler alert: this story ends with…YUMMM!

Enjoy! XO
Erika & JJ

STAY CONNECTED

 cleansimpleeats / cleansimpleeatsfit

 facebook.com/groups/cleansimpleeats

✉ hello@cleansimpleeats.com

↖ cleansimpleeats.com

RECIPE INDEX

RECIPE

INDEX

BANANAS FOSTER

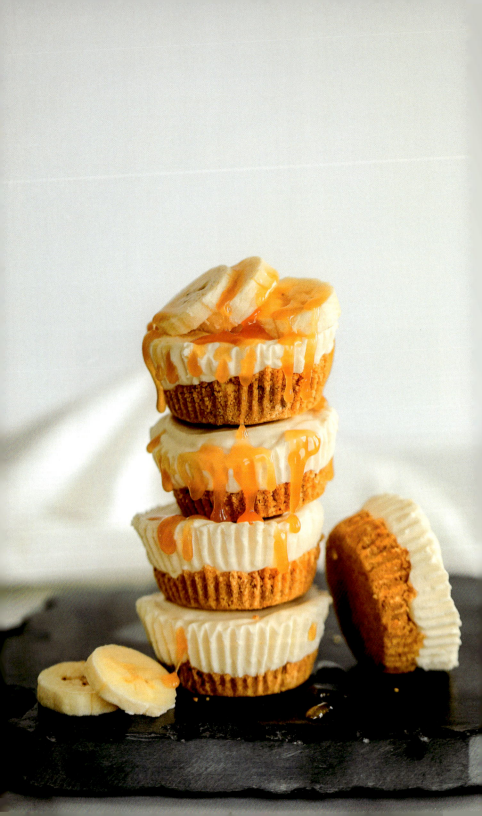

BANANA CHEESECAKE CUPS
Makes 12 servings
165 calories / 10F / 11.5C / 7P / per cup

Crust:
1 cup graham cracker crumbs
2 Tbs. grass-fed butter
1 Tbs. OffBeat Monkey Business Butter
Cheesecake:
8 oz. organic cream cheese, room temperature
2 servings (72g) CSE Bananas Foster Protein Powder
1 ½ cups Tru Whip skinny
2/3 cup plain, nonfat Greek yogurt

1. Place 12 cupcake liners in a muffin tin. Set aside.

2. Add the graham cracker crumbs to a bowl. Melt the butter. Add the melted butter and Monkey Business Butter to the bowl with the graham crackers. Stir until well combined. Weigh the mixture and divide evenly into the 12 cupcake liners. Press into the bottom and freeze.

3. Add the softened cream cheese to a mixing bowl and beat until smooth. Slowly mix in the protein powder until well combined. Add the Tru Whip and Greek yogurt; beat until smooth. Weigh the mixture and divide evenly into the cupcake liners. Using a small, rubber spatula or spoon, smooth out the top of each one.

4. Cover with foil and freeze for 2+ hours. When ready to eat, remove the cupcake liner and let thaw outside of the freezer for about 5-10 minutes. Enjoy!

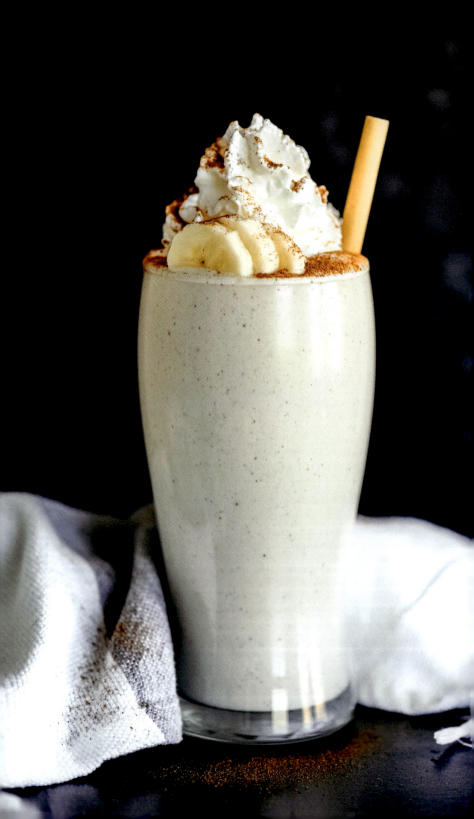

BANANAS FOSTER MILKSHAKE

Makes 1 serving
350 calories / 12F / 34C / 28P

---

1 cup unsweetened almond milk
1 serving CSE Bananas Foster Protein Powder
75g frozen banana slices
2 Tbs. low-fat cottage cheese
1 Tbs. OffBeat Cinnamon Bun Butter
 or natural almond butter
8-10 (120g) ice cubes
Topping:
2 Tbs. spray whipped cream
Dash cinnamon

1. Add all of the ingredients to a high-powered blender. Blend on high until smooth.

2. Pour into a cup. Top with whipped cream and dash of cinnamon. Enjoy!

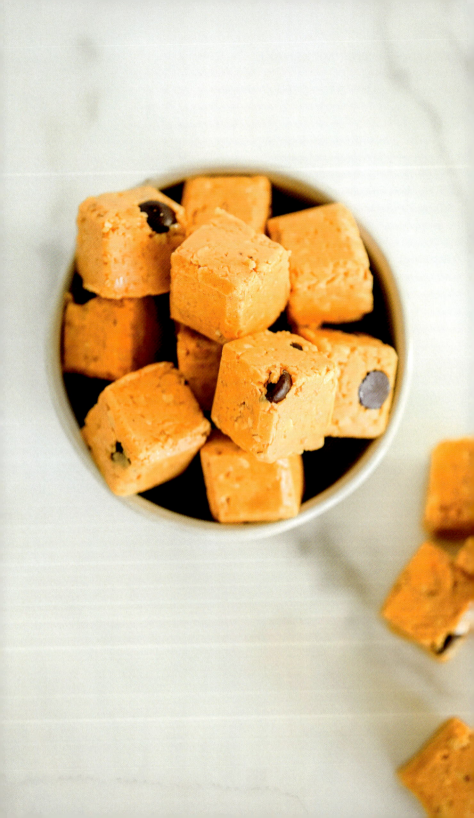

CHUNKY MONKEY BITES

Makes 26 bites / 1 bite per serving
105 calories / 5.5F / 10C / 4.5P / per bite

---

1 cup OffBeat Sweet Classic Peanut Butter
  or natural peanut butter
½ cup raw honey
2 servings CSE Bananas Foster Protein Powder
1 cup old-fashioned rolled oats
2 Tbs. dark chocolate chips
½ tsp. vanilla extract
Dash of sea salt

1. Add all the ingredients to a large bowl and mix until well combined. Works great in a Kitchen Aid Mixer!

2. Using a small cookie scoop, scoop into balls (or press into a silicone ice cube tray) and place in a container. Store in the fridge or freezer. Enjoy!

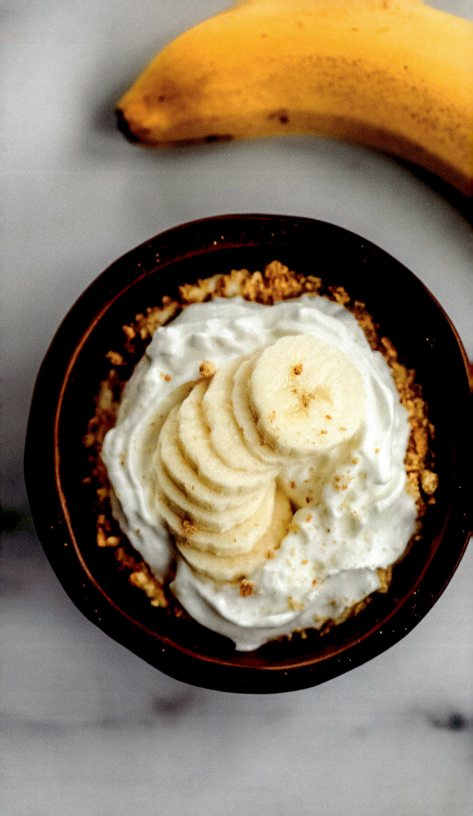

BANANA CREAM PIE PARFAIT

Makes 1 serving
210 calories / 5F / 23.5C / 18P

½ cup nonfat, plain Greek yogurt
Vanilla stevia drops, optional for sweetness
¼ serving (8g) CSE Bananas Foster Protein Powder
½ cup spray whipped cream
8g graham cracker crumbs
30g banana slices

1. Add the the yogurt, stevia and protein powder to a small bowl; mix until smooth.

2. Top with whipped cream, graham cracker crumbs and banana slices.

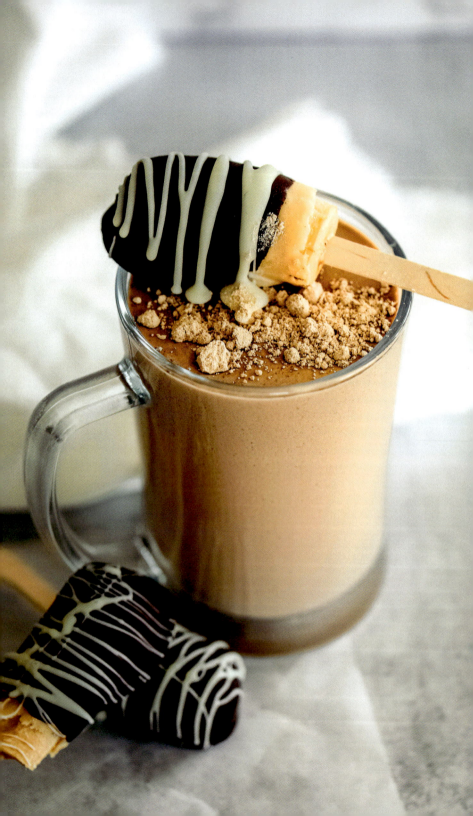

CHOCOLATE COVERED BANANA SHAKE

Makes 1 serving
220 calories / 4F / 20C / 27P

1 cup chocolate almond milk
1 serving CSE Bananas Foster Protein Powder
2 Tbs. chocolate peanut butter powder
30g frozen bananas
8-10 (130g) ice cubes

1. Add all of the ingredients to a high-powered blender. Blend on high until smooth.

2. Pour into a cup and enjoy!

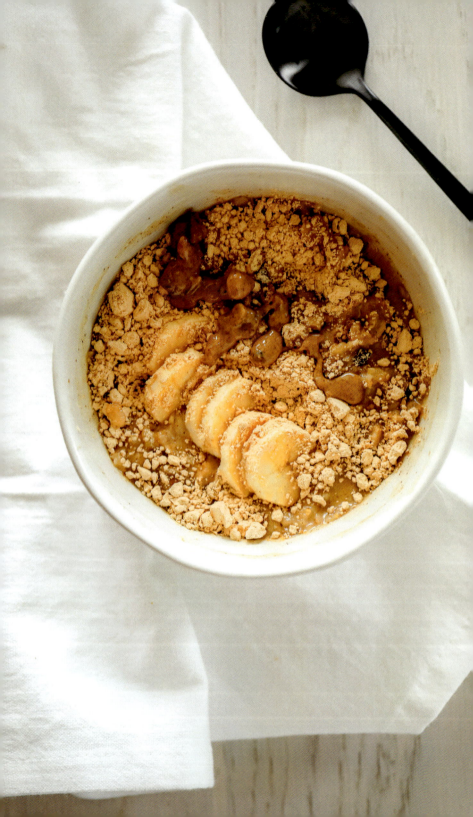

MONKEY BUSINESS OATS

Makes 1 serving
350 calories / 11F / 36C / 27P

⅓ cup old-fashioned rolled oats
½ cup water
1 Tbs. (14g) OffBeat Monkey Business Butter
   or natural peanut butter
¾ serving (27g) CSE Bananas Foster Protein Powder
20g banana slices
1 ½ Tbs. (12g) powdered peanut butter

1. Add the oats and water to a bowl. Heat in the microwave for 1.5 minutes or on the stovetop for about 5 minutes.

2. Add the nut butter and stir until smooth. Add the protein powder and stir until smooth. Top with banana slices and powdered peanut butter. Enjoy!

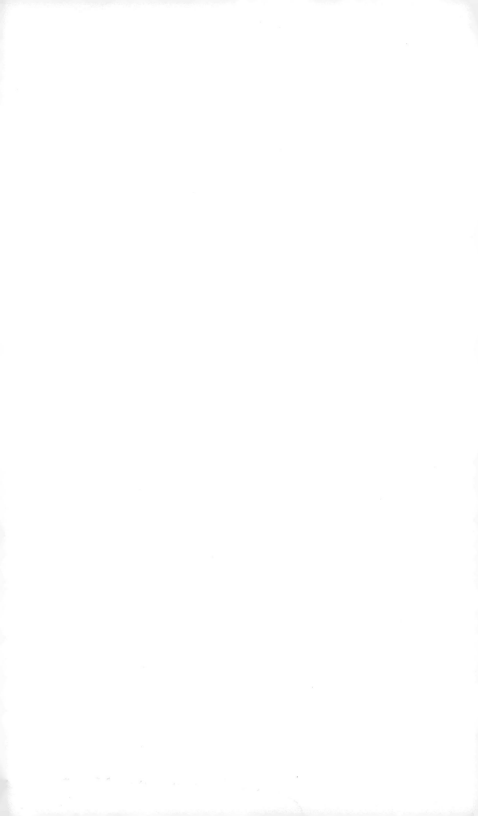

BROWNIE BATTER

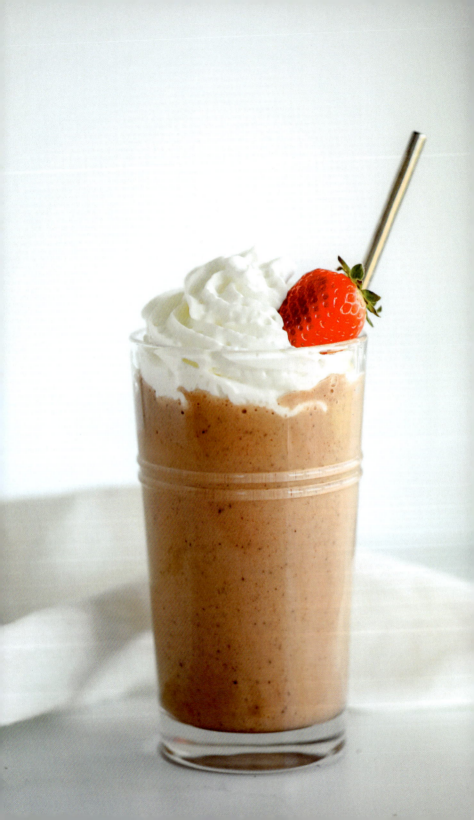

CHOCOLATE COVERED BERRY SHAKE
Makes 1 serving
215 calories / 4.5F / 21C / 22.5P

½ cup water
1 serving (34g) CSE Brownie Batter Protein Powder
1 Tbs. (16g) OffBeat Midnight Almond Coconut Butter
  or 1 Tbs. (15g) dark chocolate chips
1 serving CSE Super Berry Mix
¼ tsp. xanthan gum, optional for thickness
6-8 (120g) ice cubes
Topping:
2 Tbs. spray whipped cream

1. Add all of the ingredients to a high-powered blender. Blend on high until smooth.

2. Pour into a cup, top with whipped cream and enjoy!

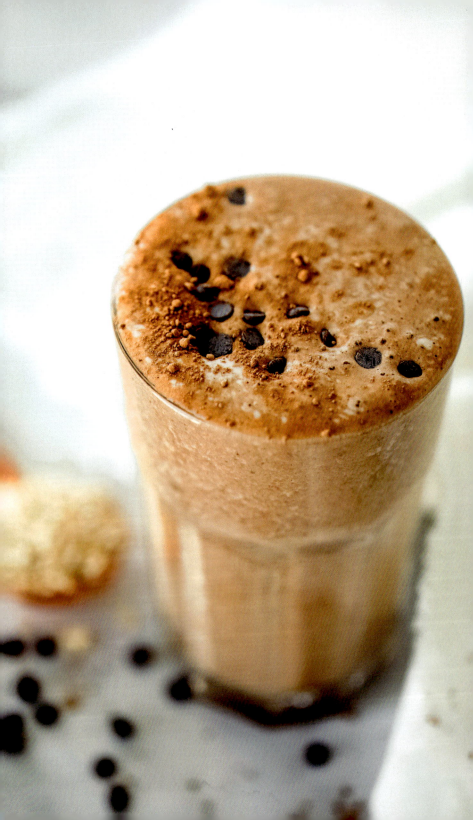

TRIPLE CHOCOLATE BROWNIE SHAKE
Makes 1 serving
330 calories / 10F / 35C / 24.5P

---

1 cup unsweetened vanilla almond milk
1 serving CSE Brownie Batter Protein Powder
30g frozen banana slices
2 Tbs. old-fashioned rolled oats
1 Tbs. cocoa powder
¼ tsp. vanilla extract
Dash sea salt
30 (15g) extra dark chocolate chips
6-8 (120g) ice cubes

1. Add all of the ingredients to a high-powered blender. Blend on high until smooth.

2. Pour into a cup and enjoy!

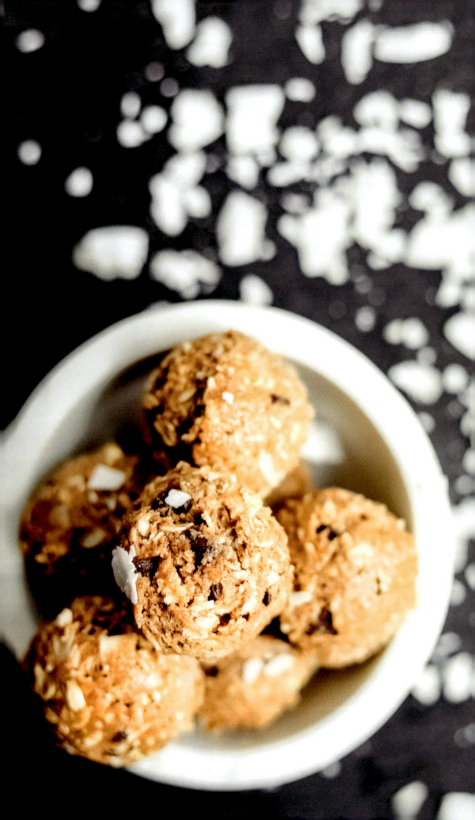

CHOCOLATE ALMOND JOY BITES

Makes 30 bites
100 calories / 5F / 10.5C / 3.5P / per bite

---

1 cup OffBeat Midnight Almond Coconut Butter
   or natural almond butter
½ cup raw honey
2 servings CSE Brownie Batter Protein Powder
½ cup unsweetened shredded coconut
2 Tbs. cocao nibs or mini chocolate chips
1 ½ cups old-fashioned rolled oats
1 tsp. vanilla extract
Dash sea salt

(Easily prepared in a Kitchen Aid Mixer)

1. Mix all ingredients together, adding the oats last, until well combined.

2. Using a small cookie scoop, scoop into balls and store in the fridge or freezer. Enjoy!

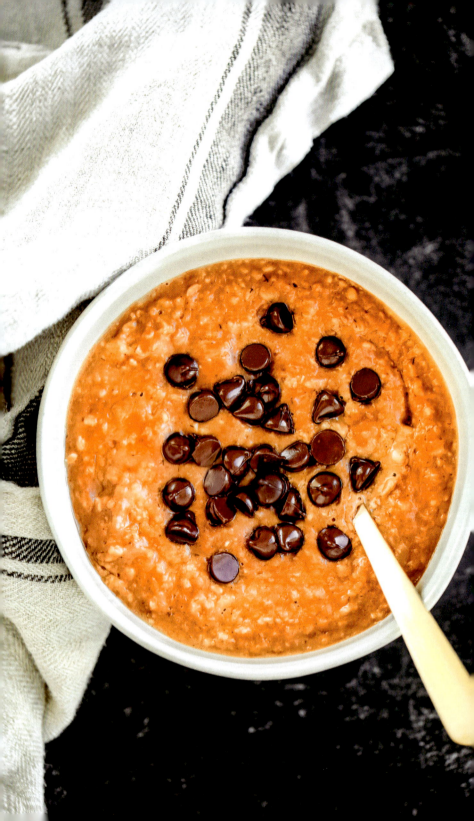

CHOCOLATE PEANUT BUTTER CUP OATMEAL
Makes 1 serving
340 calories / 11F / 32C / 27P

_____

⅓ cup old-fashioned rolled oats
⅔ cup water
3 Tbs. egg whites
2 Tbs. powdered peanut butter
2 tsp. OffBeat Sweet Classic Peanut Butter
   or natural peanut butter
½ serving CSE Chocolate Peanut Butter
   or Brownie Batter Protein Powder
15 extra dark chocolate chips

1. Mix the oats, water, egg whites and powdered peanut butter together in a bowl.

2. Microwave for 1-2 minutes or cook on the stovetop over medium heat for 5 minutes.

3. Stir in the peanut butter and let cool slightly. Stir in the protein powder and top with dark chocolate chips.

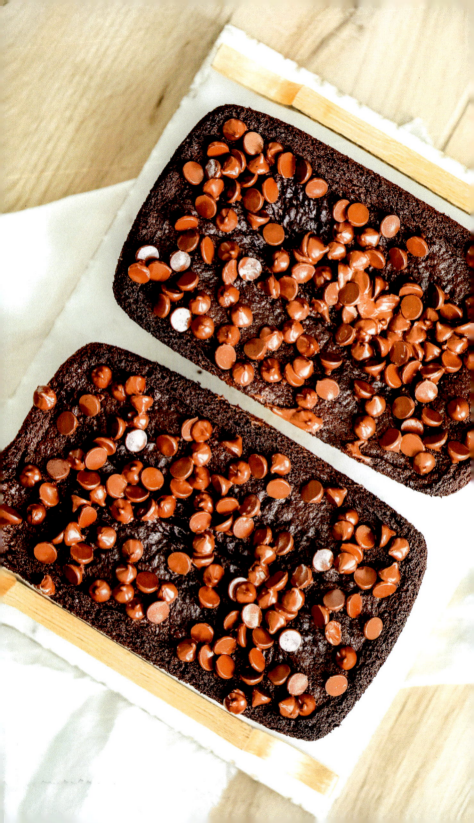

DOUBLE CHOCOLATE BANANA BREAD
Makes 1 loaf / 10 slices
240 calories / 10.5F / 35C / 7.5P / per slice

3 ripe bananas
½ cup unsweetened applesauce
½ cup raw honey
¼ cup melted coconut oil
1 large egg
1 tsp. vanilla extract
1 cup CSE Vanilla Pancake & Waffle Mix
1 serving CSE Brownie Batter Protein Powder
⅓ cup cocoa powder
½ tsp. baking soda
½ tsp baking powder
½ tsp. sea salt
½ cup dark chocolate chips

1. Preheat the oven to 350 degrees.

2. Mash the bananas in a large bowl. Beat in the applesauce, honey and melted coconut oil. Add the egg and vanilla; mix well.

3. In a separate bowl, combine the CSE Pancake & Waffle Mix, protein powder, cocoa powder, baking soda, baking powder and sea salt. Add the dry ingredients to the wet ingredients. Mix until just combined.

4. Pour into a greased 9x5 inch, glass loaf pan and sprinkle with the chocolate chips. Bake for 50-55 minutes, then let cool. Remove from the pan and drizzle with extra melted chocolate, if desired. Store extras in the fridge or freezer.

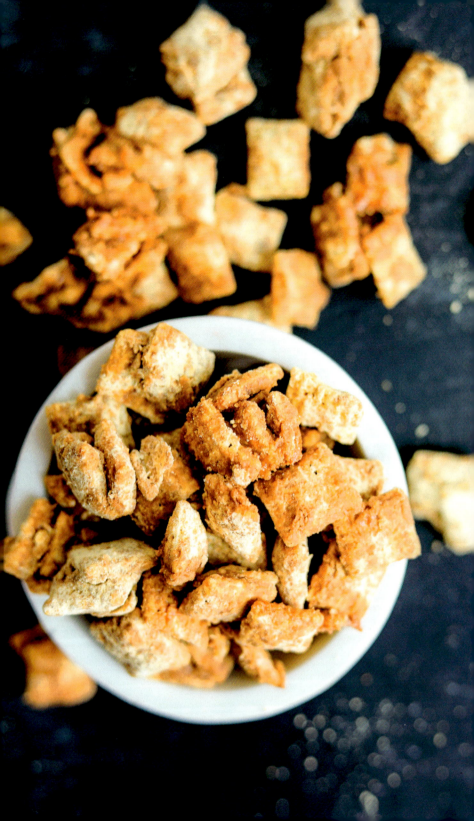

BROWNIE BATTER BUDDIES

Makes 16 servings / ½ cup (45g) per serving
185 calories / 5F / 29C / 7P / per serving

¾ cup raw honey
½ cup OffBeat Sweet Classic Peanut Butter, Buckeye Brownie
    Peanut Butter, or natural peanut butter
1 tsp. vanilla extract
1 serving CSE Brownie Batter or Chocolate Peanut Butter
    Protein Powder
1 Tbs. cocoa powder
8 cups Rice Chex cereal
1 cup powdered peanut butter

1. In a small saucepan melt together the honey, peanut butter and vanilla over low heat. Stir until melted together and smooth, then remove from heat. Stir in the protein powder and cocoa powder.

2. Place Chex cereal into a large bowl. Pour the hot mixture over the top and gently stir until the cereal is well-coated.

3. Pour the powdered peanut butter over the top and stir until well-coated. Store any extras in the fridge. Enjoy!

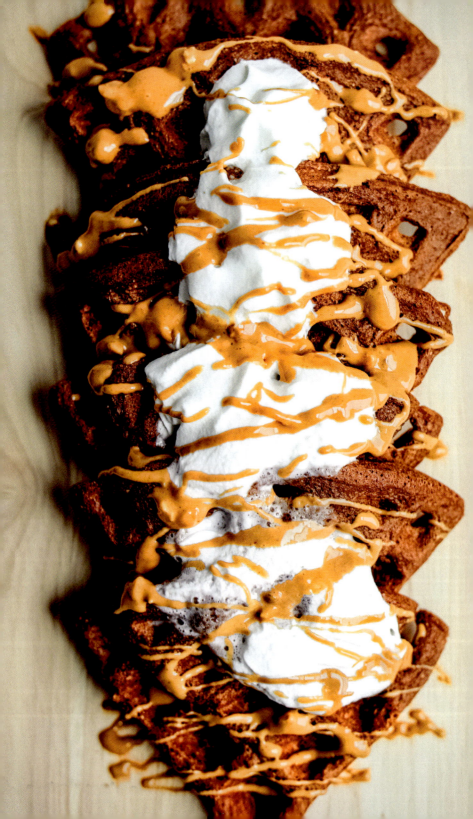

CHOCOLATE WAFFLES

Makes 4 servings
350 calories / 12F / 36C / 25.5P / per serving

---

1 ¾ cup CSE Vanilla Pancake & Waffle Mix
1 serving CSE Brownie Batter Protein Powder
1 Tbs. cocoa powder
1 ¼ cups water
2 large eggs
40g mashed banana

Toppings per serving:
1 Tbs. OffBeat Sweet Classic, Buckeye Brownie Peanut Butter
   or natural peanut butter
2 Tbs. spray whipped cream
Zero calorie syrup of choice

1. Preheat waffle iron.

2. In a medium-sized bowl, mix together the CSE Pancake & Waffle Mix, protein powder, cocoa powder, water, eggs, and banana. Stir together until well combined.

3. Spray the waffle iron with cooking spray. Pour the batter into the waffle iron. Repeat with the remaining batter. Weigh the waffles and divide the weight by four to get the amount needed to fill one serving.

3. Top each serving with one tablespoon of peanut butter, two tablespoons of whipped cream and syrup. Enjoy!

CAKE
BATTER

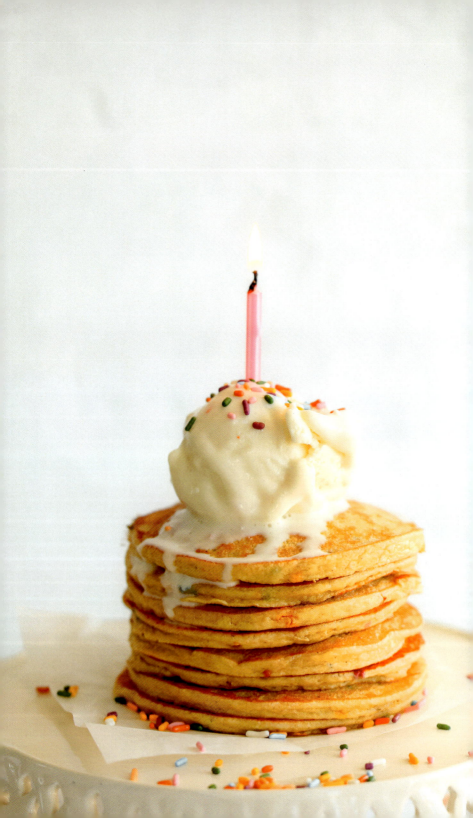

BIRTHDAY CAKES & ICE CREAM
Makes 4 servings
260 calories / 9F / 25.5C / 19P / per serving

½ cup unsweetened almond milk
¼ cup nonfat, plain Greek yogurt
2 large eggs
1 Tbs. coconut oil
½ tsp. vanilla extract
1 cup old-fashioned rolled oats
2 servings CSE Cake Batter Protein Powder
1 tsp. baking powder
1 Tbs. rainbow sprinkles
Topping per serving:
30g Birthday Cake or Vanilla high-protein ice cream

1. Add all of the ingredients, except for the sprinkles and ice cream, to a blender. Blend on high until smooth. Add the sprinkles and stir into the batter until well combined.

2. Heat a griddle to medium heat. Once hot, spray with cooking spray and add ¼ cup of the batter to the griddle for each pancake. Once small bubbles form on the outside of the pancakes, flip and cook until golden brown on both sides. Makes about 8 pancakes. Divide the pancakes by 4 to get the amount needed to fill one serving.

3. Top each serving of pancakes with ice cream (plus a candle if you're feeling fancy) and enjoy!

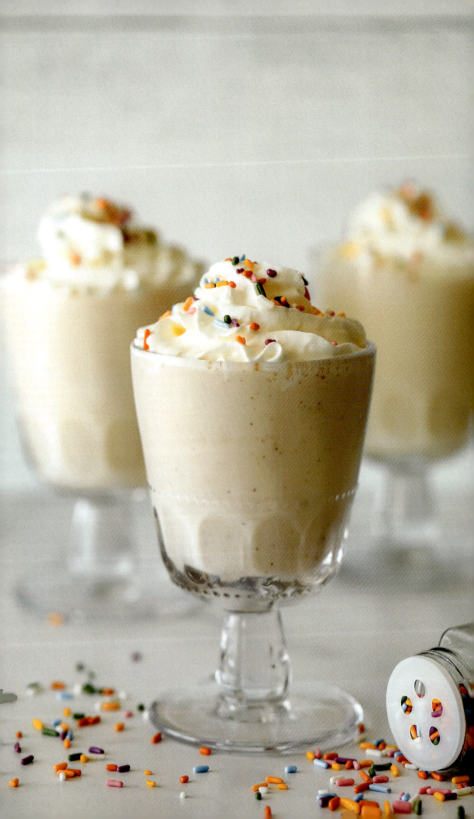

BIRTHDAY CAKE MILKSHAKE
Makes 1 serving
245 calories / 9F / 23C / 17.5P

___

¾ cup unsweetened almond milk
½ serving CSE Birthday Cake Protein Powder
   or CSE Simply Vanilla Protein Powder
½ cup Birthday Cake or Vanilla high-protein ice cream
½ Tbs. (7g) OffBeat Aloha, Salted Caramel, Lemon Coconut Bliss
   or natural almond butter
8-10 (120g) ice cubes
Topping:
2 Tbs. spray whipped cream
1 tsp. sprinkles

1. Add all of the ingredients to a high-powered blender. Blend on high until smooth.

2. Pour into a cup. Top with whipped cream and sprinkles. Enjoy!

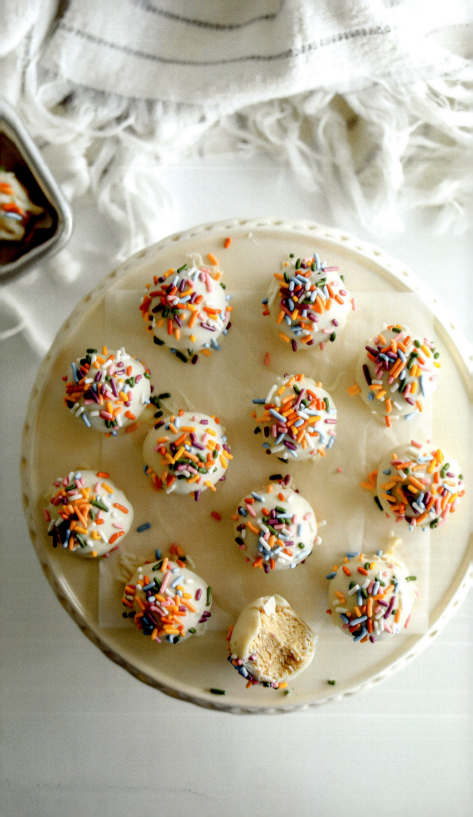

LEMON CAKE POPS

Makes 26 bites / 1 cake pop per serving
150 calories / 9.5F / 12C / 4P / per serving

---

12 oz. OffBeat Lemon Coconut Bliss Butter
  or natural almond butter
½ cup raw honey
2 servings CSE Cake Batter Protein Powder
1 cup almond flour
Pinch sea salt
Dash vanilla extract
Toppings:
50g white chocolate chips
1 Tbs. rainbow sprinkles

1. Add the nut butter, honey, protein powder, almond lour, sea salt and vanilla extract to a bowl. Mix until well combined. Place in the fridge to harden for 30 minutes.

2. Remove from the fridge. Using a small cookie scoop, scoop into balls and place on a baking sheet lined with parchment paper. Return to the fridge while making the topping.

3. Add the white chocolate chips to a microwave safe bowl. Heat for 30 seconds at a time until completely melted. Drizzle the melted chocolate over one ball at a time and immediately add the sprinkles, so they will stick to the chocolate before it hardens. Store in the fridge. Enjoy!

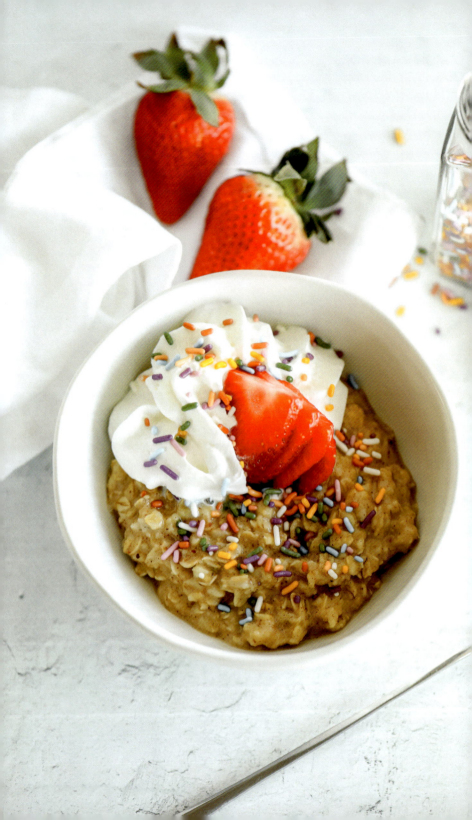

CONFETTI CAKE OATMEAL

Makes 1 serving
325 calories / 10.5F / 31C / 26P

⅓ cup old-fashioned rolled oats
½ cup water
3 Tbs. (47g) liquid egg whites
1 Tbs. (14g) OffBeat Salted Caramel Butter
   or natural almond butter
¾ serving (24g) CSE Cake Batter Protein Powder
Toppings:
2 Tbs. spray whipped cream
40g strawberries
½ tsp. rainbow sprinkles

1. Add the oats, water and egg whites to a bowl. Microwave for 1.5 minutes or cook in a pot on the stovetop for about 5 minutes, stirring halfway through.

2. Add the nut butter and stir until well combined. Let cool for 1-2 minutes, then add the protein powder and stir until dissolved. Top with whipped cream, strawberries and sprinkles. Enjoy!

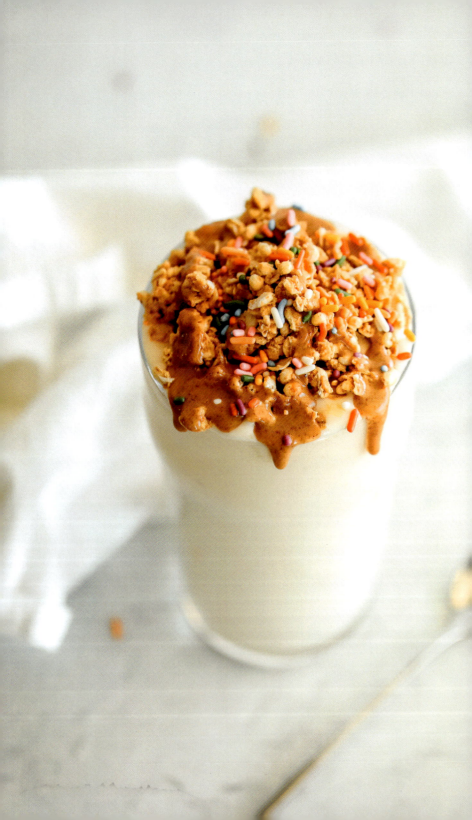

CAKE BATTER BLISS SHAKE

Makes 1 serving
350 calories / 12F / 34C / 27P

---

1 cup unsweetened vanilla almond milk
1 serving CSE Cake Batter Protein Powder
60g frozen banana slices
6-8 (120g) ice cubes
Toppings:
17g Kashi Coconut Almond Crunch Cereal
1 Tbs. OffBeat Salted Caramel Butter
   or natural almond butter
½ tsp. rainbow sprinkles

1. Add the almond milk, protein powder, bananas and ice to a blender. Blend on high until smooth. Pour into a cup.

2. Top with cereal, Salted Caramel Butter and sprinkles. Mix in and enjoy with a spoon!

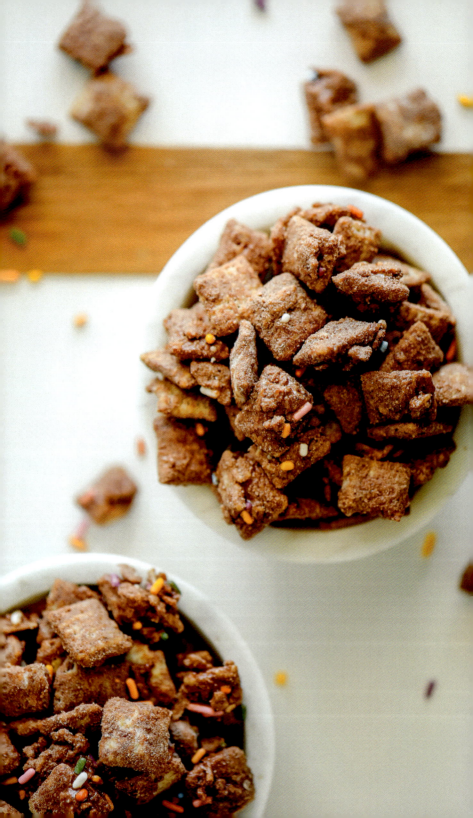

MUDDY CAKE BUDDIES

Makes 6 servings
250 calories / 12F / 29C / 6P / per serving

---

3 cups Vanilla Chex Cereal
1 serving CSE Cake Batter Protein Powder
1 Tbs. rainbow sprinkles
1 Tbs. grass-fed butter
3 Tbs. OffBeat Butters Salted Caramel Butter
   or natural almond butter
⅓ cup (65g) semi-sweet chocolate chips

1. Pour the Chex cereal into a bowl. Set aside.

2. Combine the protein powder and sprinkles in a large Ziploc bag. Set aside.

3. Melt the butter in a small saucepan over low heat. Once melted, add the nut butter and chocolate chips. Stir until melted and smooth.

4. Pour the melted chocolate mixture over the cereal and toss until well coated. Pour the chocolate coated cereal into the Ziploc bag with the protein powder and sprinkles. Shake until well coated.

5. Weigh the entire mix and divide by six to get the amount needed to fill one serving. Enjoy!

CARAMEL TOFFEE

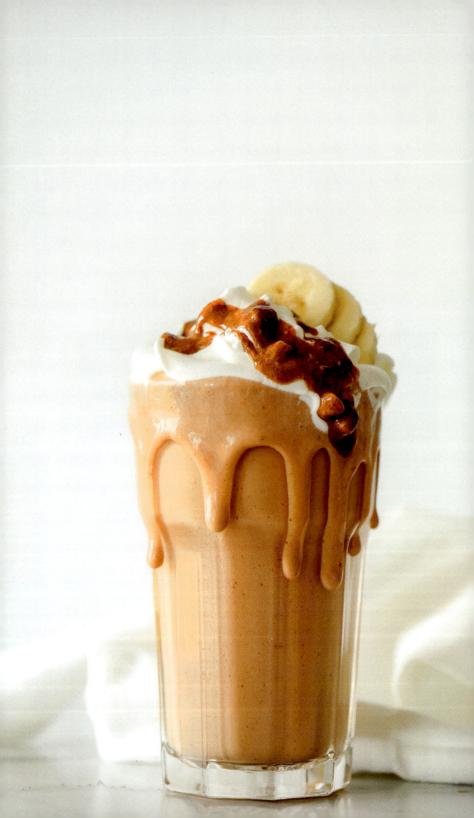

CHOCOLATE CARAMEL BANANA SHAKE

Makes 1 serving
350 calories / 13.5F / 33C / 27P / per serving

---

1 cup unsweetened almond milk
1 serving CSE Caramel Toffee Protein Powder
1 Tbs. (14g) OffBeat Crunchy Almond Toffee Butter
    Salted Caramel Butter, or natural almond butter
80g frozen banana slices
1 Tbs. low-fat cottage cheese
1 Tbs. cocoa powder
6-8 (120g) ice cubes
Topping:
2 Tbs. spray whipped cream

1. Add all of the ingredients to a high-powered blender. Blend on high until smooth.

2. Pour into a cup and top with whipped cream. Enjoy!

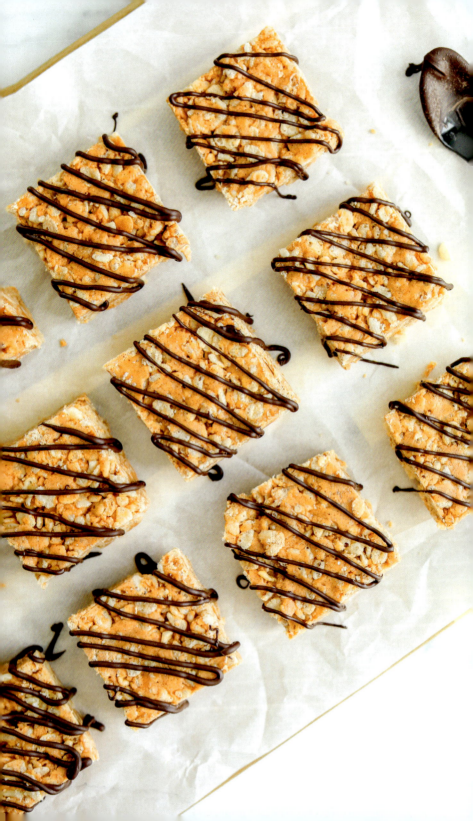

CRISPY CARAMEL BUTTERSCOTCH BARS

Makes 18 bars / 1 bar per serving
225 calories / 12.5F / 23C / 5P / per bar

Bars:

12 oz. OffBeat Salted Caramel Butter
   or natural almond butter
½ cup raw honey
2 Tbs. unsweetened almond milk
½ cup butterscotch chips
1 serving CSE Caramel Toffee Protein Powder
3 ¾ cups crispy rice cereal

Topping:

¼ cup dark chocolate chips

1. Add the nut butter, honey, almond milk and butterscotch chips to a saucepan over low/medium heat. Stir until the butterscotch chips are melted and the mixture is smooth. Remove from heat and stir in the protein powder. Mix until well combined.

2. Pour the cereal into a large bowl and top with the caramel butterscotch mixture. Beat together until the ingredients are well combined. Press into a greased 9x13 pan. Store in the fridge until hardened and cool.

3. Place the chocolate chips in a small bowl. Microwave for 1-2 minutes or until melted and smooth, stirring every 30 seconds.

4. Remove the bars from the 9x13 pan onto a cutting board. Cut into 18 squares. Drizzle the chocolate over the top of the bars. Let the chocolate harden and enjoy! Store leftovers in the fridge.

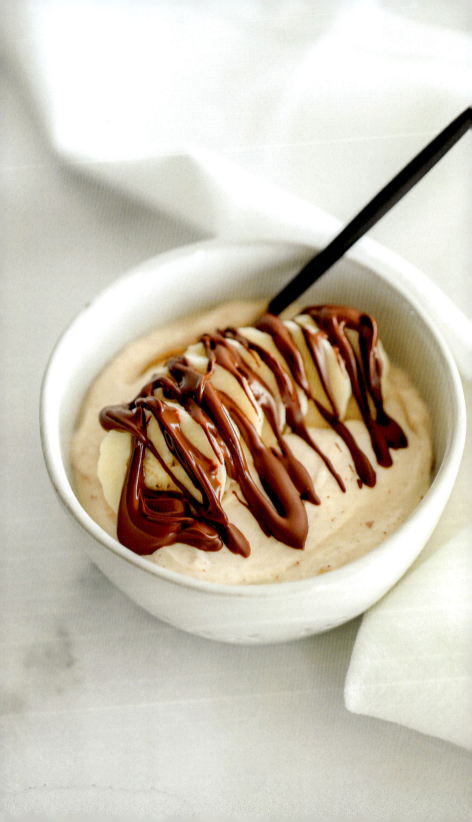

CHOCOLATE CARAMEL PROTEIN PARFAIT
Makes 1 serving
225 calories / 7.5F / 22.5C / 20.5P / per serving

½ cup nonfat, plain Greek yogurt
1 Tbs. unsweetened almond milk
10g CSE Caramel Toffee Protein Powder
½ Tbs. (7g) OffBeat Crunchy Almond Toffee Butter
  or natural almond butter
45g bananas
  or 90g apples
2 tsp. mini chocolate chips

1. Add the Greek yogurt, almond milk, protein powder and OffBeat Butter to a bowl. Stir until smooth.

2. Slice up a banana or apple. Top with sliced bananas or apples and mini chocolate chips. Enjoy!

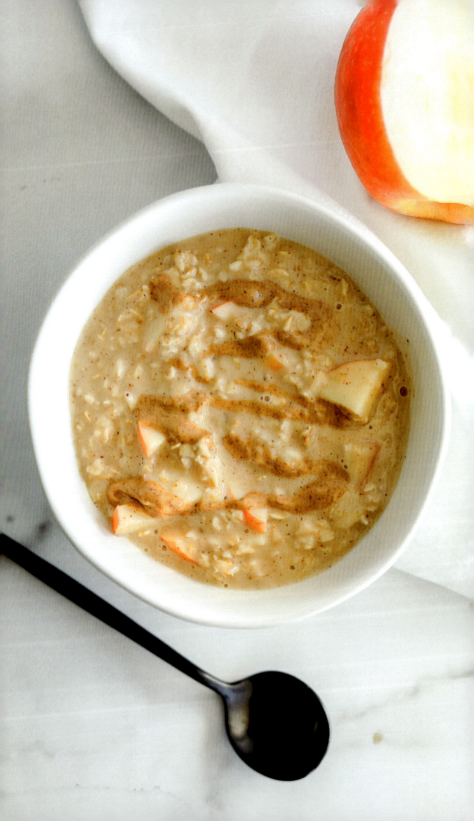

DOUBLE CARAMEL APPLE OATMEAL
Makes 1 serving
340 calories / 10F / 37C / 26P per serving

⅓ cup old-fashioned rolled oats
½ cup water
3 Tbs. (46g) liquid egg whites
50g chopped apples
1 Tbs. (14g) OffBeat Salted Caramel Butter
   or natural almond butter
¾ serving (24g) CSE Caramel Toffee Protein Powder
Dash of cinnamon

1. Add the oats, water, egg whites and chopped apples to a bowl.

2. Microwave for 1.5 minutes or cook on the stovetop for 5 minutes. Stir in the nut butter and the protein powder.

3. Top with cinnamon. Enjoy!

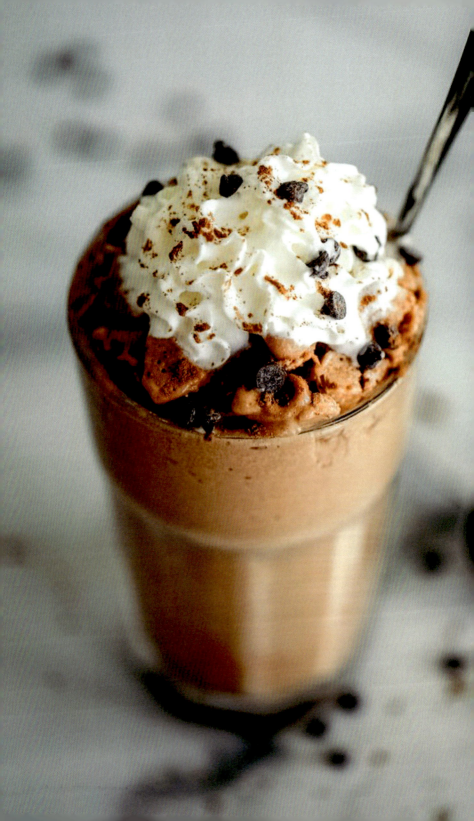

CHOCOLATE CARAMEL TOFFEE MILKSHAKE

Makes 1 serving
230 calories / 7F / 19C / 22P / per serving

---

1 cup unsweetened vanilla almond milk
1 serving CSE Caramel Toffee Protein Powder
1 Tbs. cocoa powder
¼ tsp. xanthan gum
8-10 (140g) ice cubes
Topping:
2 Tbs. spray whipped cream topping
2 tsp. mini chocolate chips

1. Add all of the shake ingredients to a high-powered blender. Blend on high until smooth.

2. Pour into cup and add toppings. Milkshake should be thick. Enjoy with a spoon!

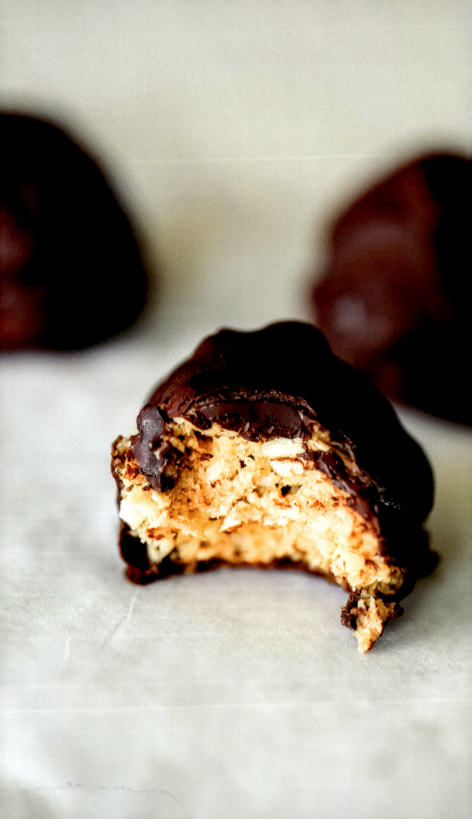

SNICKERS POWER BITES

Makes 28 servings
110 calories / 5.5F / 11C / 4P / per bite

---

1 cup OffBeat Candy Bar Butter, Sweet Classic Peanut Butter, Salted Caramel Butter or natural peanut butter.
½ cup raw honey
1 serving CSE Caramel Toffee Protein Powder
½ tsp. vanilla extract
Dash sea salt
1 ½ cups old-fashioned rolled oats
Cocoa Dusting:
¼ cup cocoa powder
Chocolate Coating:
120g dark chocolate chips

1. Add all of the ingredients to a large bowl and mix until well combined.

2. Using a small cookie scoop, scoop into balls.

3. If using the Cocoa Dusting method (100 calories per ball): Add the cocoa powder to a bowl and roll each ball into it. Place in a container and store in the fridge or freezer.

4. If using the Chocolate Coating method (110 calories per ball): Add the chocolate chips to a microwave safe bowl. Microwave for 1-2 minutes or until melted and smooth, stirring every 30 seconds.

5. Roll each ball in the chocolate coating and scoop out using a fork or slotted spoon. Tap on bowl to remove excess chocolate then place on a baking sheet lined with parchment paper. Place in the fridge or freezer to allow the chocolate coating to set. Transfer to a container and store in the fridge or freezer.

CHOCOLATE PEANUT BUTTER

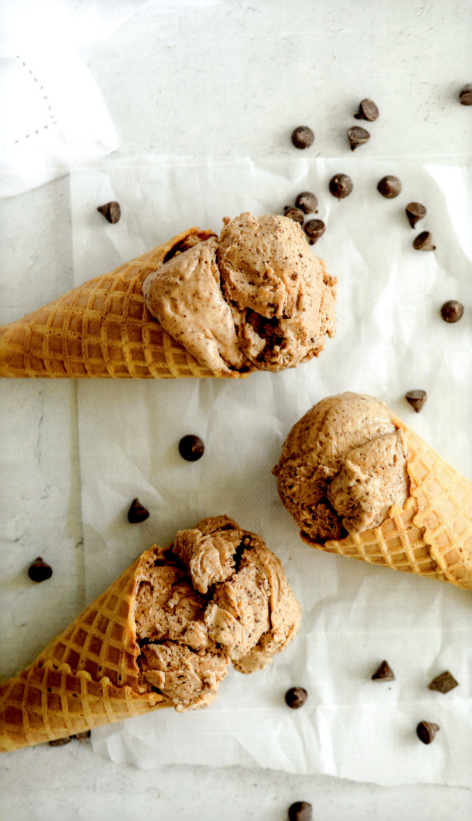

CHOCOLATE SPECKLED PB ICE CREAM

Makes 4 servings
300 calories / 11.5F / 35C / 15P / per serving

400g frozen banana slices
2 servings CSE Chocolate Peanut Butter Protein Powder
¼ cup OffBeat Sweet Classic, Buckeye Brownie Peanut Butter
   or natural peanut butter
¼ cup unsweetened almond milk
3 Tbs. (45g) dark chocolate chips

1. Add all of the ingredients to a Blendtec, Vitamix or food proces-
sor. Blend until thick and smooth. Scrape down the sides and stir in
between blending, if needed.

2. Pour into a loaf pan lined with parchment paper. Freeze for 2+
hours. Use an ice cream scoop to serve the ice cream. Scoop into a
bowl or a cone.

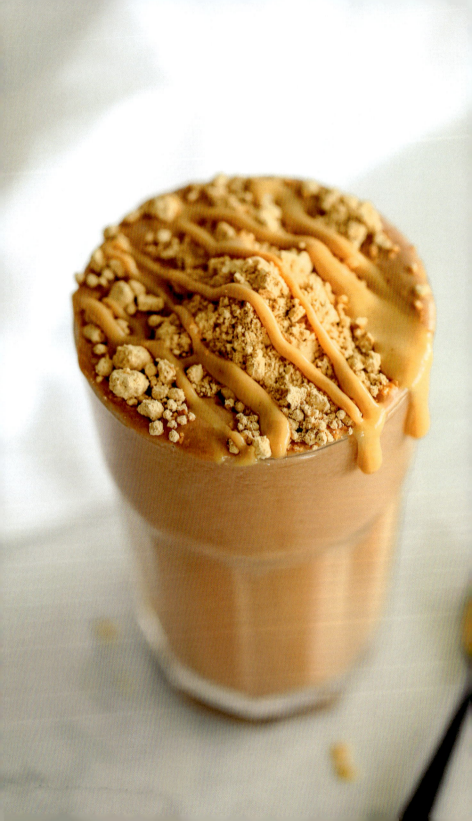

CHOCOLATE PEANUT BUTTER CUP SHAKE

Makes 1 serving
345 calories / 11F / 32C / 29.5P

---

1 cup unsweetened vanilla almond milk
1 serving CSE Chocolate Peanut Butter Protein Powder
1 Tbs. cocoa powder
14g OffBeat Sweet Classic Peanut Butter
   or natural peanut butter
60g frozen bananas
6-8 (120g) ice cubes
Topping:
1 Tbs. powdered peanut butter

1. Add all of the shake ingredients to a high-powered blender. Blend until smooth.

2. Pour into a cup. Top with powdered peanut butter and lightly fold into the shake. Enjoy!

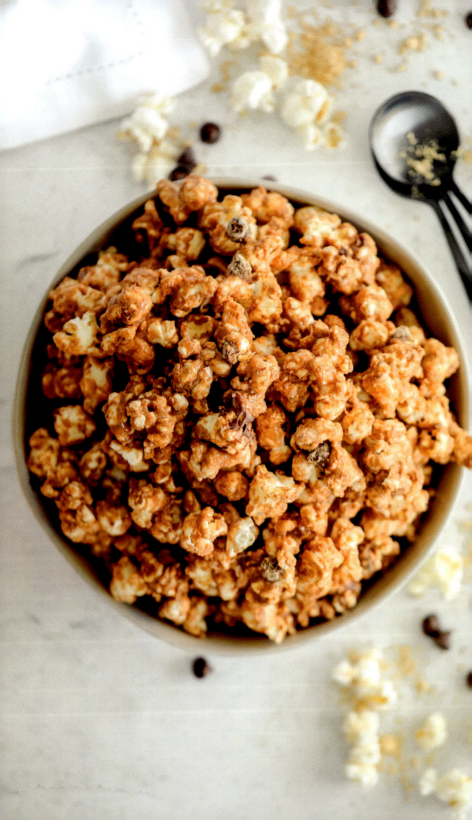

PEANUT BUTTER CUP POPCORN

Makes 8 servings / about 85g per serving
400 calories / 19.5F / 42.5C / 14P / per serving

---

12 (72g) cups air popped popcorn
1 cup (8 oz.) OffBeat Sweet Classic Peanut Butter
   or natural peanut butter
¾ (6 oz.) cup raw honey
2 Tbs. grass-fed butter
1 tsp. vanilla extract
Pinch sea salt
1 Tbs. cocoa powder
1 serving CSE Chocolate Peanut Butter Protein Powder

Topping:
60g dark chocolate chips
¼ (32g) cup powdered peanut butter
1 serving CSE Chocolate Peanut Butter Protein Powder

1. Pop the popcorn kernels (about ⅓ cup) into a large bowl. Remove all unpopped kernels from the bowl. Set aside.

2. Add the peanut butter, honey, butter and vanilla to a small sauce pan over low/medium heat. Whisk until well combined and melted down. Remove from heat.

3. Add the sea salt, cocoa powder and protein powder to the pot with the peanut butter mixture. Stir until combined. Pour over the top of the popcorn while the sauce is still warm and stir until the popcorn is well coated.

4. Sprinkle the dark chocolate chips, powdered peanut butter and protein powder over the top of the popcorn. Stir until the popcorn is well coated and all the dry powder is incorporated. Weigh the entire batch and divide by eight to get the amount needed for one serving. Enjoy!

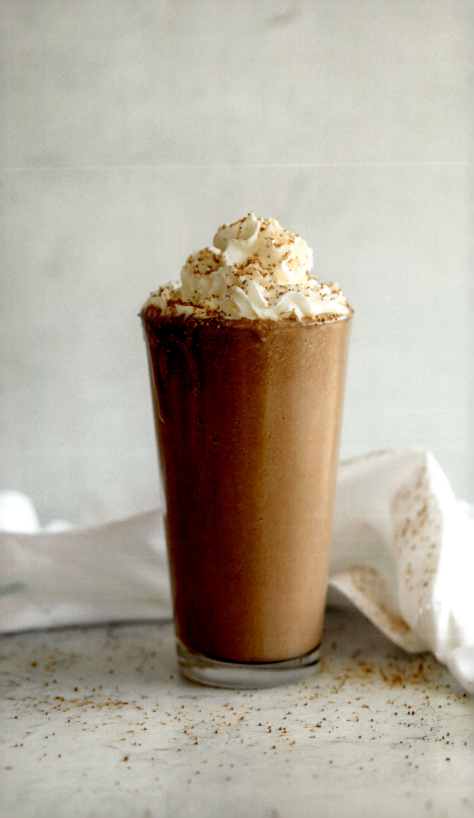

DARK CHOCOLATE PB SHAKE

Makes 1 serving
240 calories / 6F / 26C / 22.5P

---

1 cup dark chocolate almond milk
1 serving CSE Chocolate Peanut Butter Protein Powder
½ Tbs. OffBeat Sweet Classic Peanut Butter
   or natural peanut butter
6-8 (120g) ice cubes

1. Add all of the ingredients to a high-powered blender. Blend until smooth.

2. Pour into a cup. Enjoy!

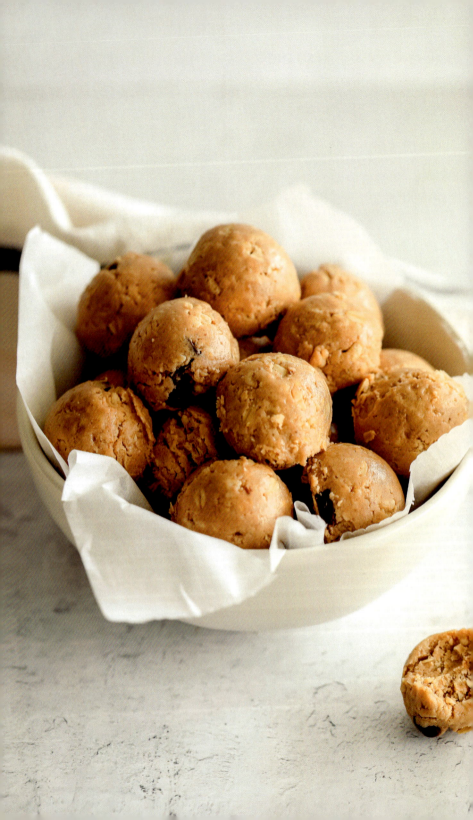

CRISPY CHOCOLATE PB BITES
Makes 25 / 1 bite per serving
100 calories / 5F / 10C / 4P / per bite

---

1 cup OffBeat Sweet Classic Peanut Butter
    or natural peanut butter
½ cup raw honey
2 servings CSE Chocolate Peanut Butter Protein Powder
Pinch of sea salt
1 tsp. vanilla extract
1 cup old-fashioned rolled oats
1 cup crispy rice cereal
2 Tbs. (30g) mini dark chocolate chips

1. Add the peanut butter, honey, protein powder, salt and vanilla to a large mixing bowl. Mix until well combined.

2. Add in the remaining ingredients and mix well.

3. Using a small cookie scoop, scoop the dough into balls and place in a container. Store in the fridge or freezer. Enjoy!

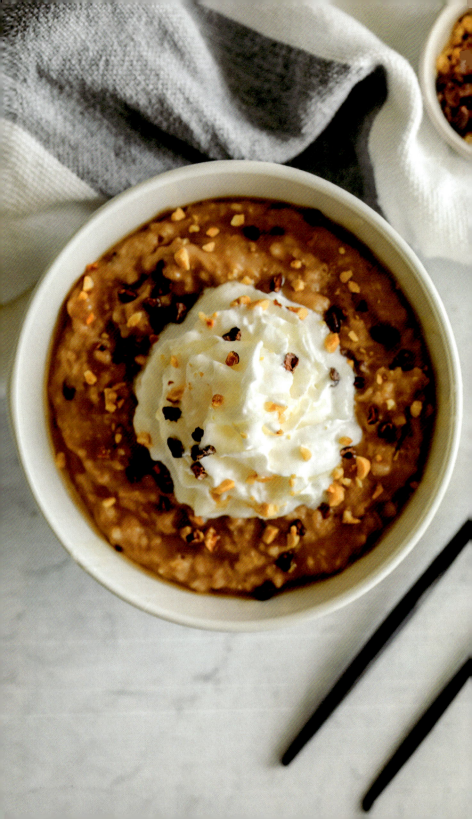

CANDY BAR OATS

Makes 1 serving
355 calories / 13F / 32C / 28P

⅓ cup old-fashioned rolled oats
½ cup water
1 Tbs. OffBeat Candy Bar Peanut Butter
   or natural peanut butter
1 serving CSE Chocolate Peanut Butter Protein Powder
1 Tbs. spray whipped cream
½ (4g) Tbs. cacao nibs or dark chocolate chips
½ (4g) Tbs. chopped peanuts
½ tsp. honey

1. Add the rolled oats and water to a bowl. Microwave on high for 1½ minutes.

2. Stir in the Candy Bar Butter and let cool a bit. Stir in protein powder until well combined.

3. Top with spray whipped cream, nibs, chopped peanuts and a drizzle of honey. Enjoy!

CINNAMON ROLL

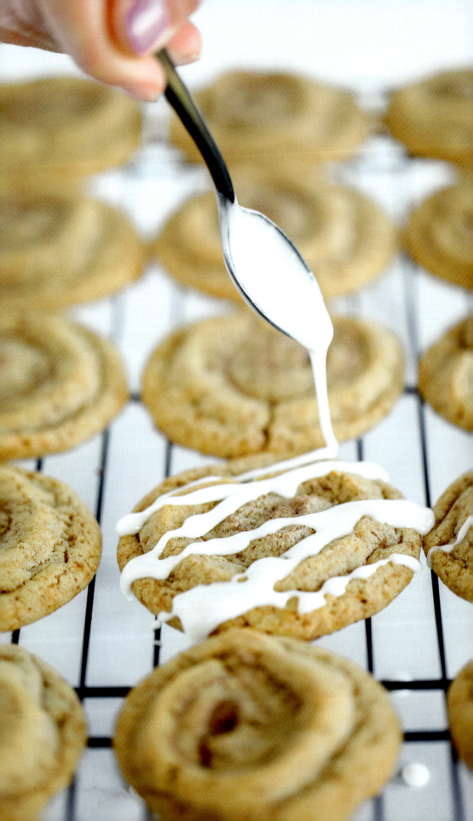

CINNAMON ROLL COOKIES

Makes 16 cookies
195 calories / 8F / 28C / 4P / per cookie

½ cup grass-fed butter
¼ cup organic cane sugar
½ cup coconut sugar
1 large egg
½ tsp. vanilla extract
1 ½ cups (180g) whole wheat pastry flour
1 serving CSE Cinnamon Roll Protein Powder
½ tsp. baking soda
¼ tsp. sea salt
Filling:
¼ cup (56g) OffBeat Cinnamon Bun Butter
   or natural almond butter
Icing:
½ cup organic powdered sugar
1 Tbs. liquid egg whites

1. Preheat the oven to 350 degrees.

2. Add the softened butter, cane sugar and coconut sugar to a mixing bowl. Mix together until smooth. Add the egg and vanilla, beat together until smooth.

3. In a separate bowl add the flour, protein powder, baking soda and sea salt. Stir until incorporated. Add the dry to the wet ingredients and mix until just combined.

4. Lay a large piece of parchment paper out on the counter. Sprinkle a little flour over the top. Place the large ball of dough on the parchment paper. Using a floured rolling pin, roll the dough out into a large rectangle. Spread the OffBeat Butter evenly over the dough. Carefully roll the dough up lengthwise like a cinnamon roll. Once completely rolled up, gently slice into 16 equal sized cookies. Place each cookie on a baking sheet lined with parchment paper and bake for 8-9 minutes. Let cool for a few minutes and then transfer to a cooling rack.

5. Make the icing by adding the powdered sugar and egg whites to a small bowl. Whisk together until well combined and smooth. Drizzle over the cooled cookies.

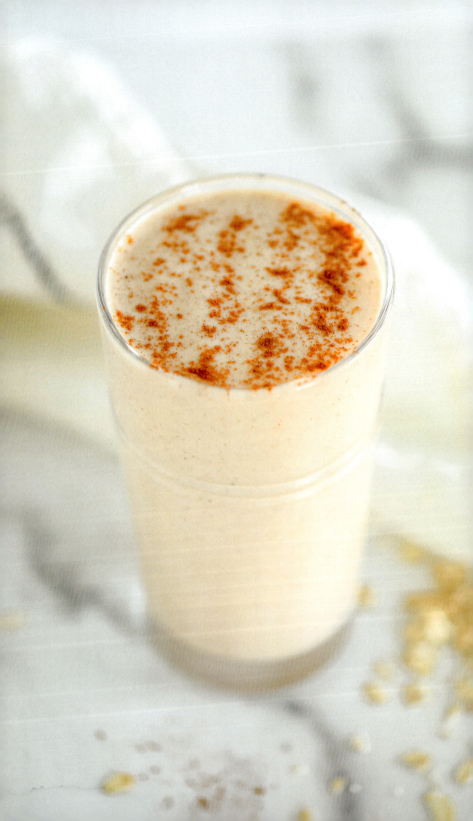

CINNAMON BUN SHAKE

Makes 1 serving
335 calories / 13F / 34.5C / 27P

1 cup unsweetened almond milk
¼ cup low-fat cottage cheese
¾ serving (25g) CSE Cinnamon Roll Protein Powder
50g frozen bananas slices
2 Tbs. old-fashioned rolled oats
1 Tbs. OffBeat Cinnamon Bun Butter
   or natural almond butter
½ tsp. cinnamon
6-8 (120g) ice cubes

1. Add all of the ingredients to a high-powered blender. Blend on high until smooth.

2. Pour into a cup. Enjoy!

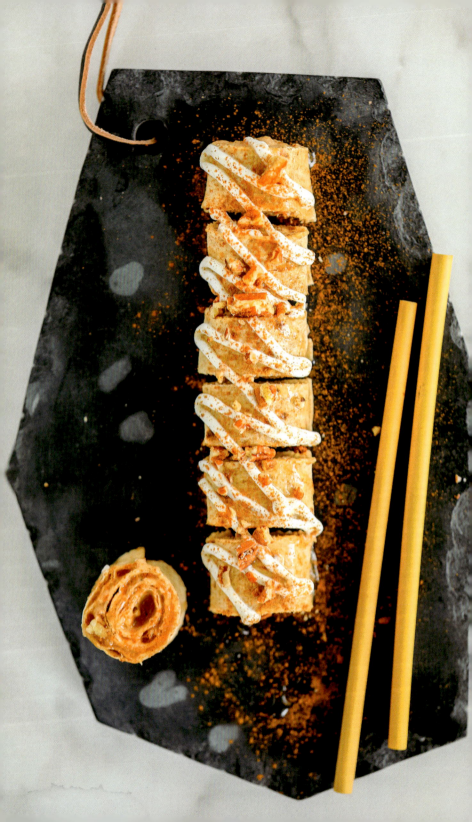

CINNAMON ROLL'D SUSHI

Makes 1 serving
350 calories / 13F / 37C / 26.5P

---

1 Joseph's Lavash Bread
¼ cup nonfat, plain Greek yogurt, divided
1 Tbs. OffBeat Cinnamon Bun Butter
   or natural almond butter
⅔ serving (21g) CSE Cinnamon Roll Protein Powder
 Vanilla stevia drops, optional
1 Tbs. raw honey
1 Tbs. (7g) chopped pecans

1. Add 3 Tbs. Greek yogurt, Cinnamon Bun Butter and Cinnamon Roll Protein Powder to a small bowl. Mix until smooth.

2. Lay the Lavash out flat on a plate. Add the yogurt mixture to the center and spread out evenly to cover the wrap.

3. Roll the wrap up tight, lengthwise and cut into one inch slices to create your "sushi".

4. Add the honey, remaining 1 Tbs. Greek yogurt and stevia (if desired) to a small bowl. Mix until smooth. Drizzle over the top of the sushi rolls and garnish with chopped pecans. Enjoy!

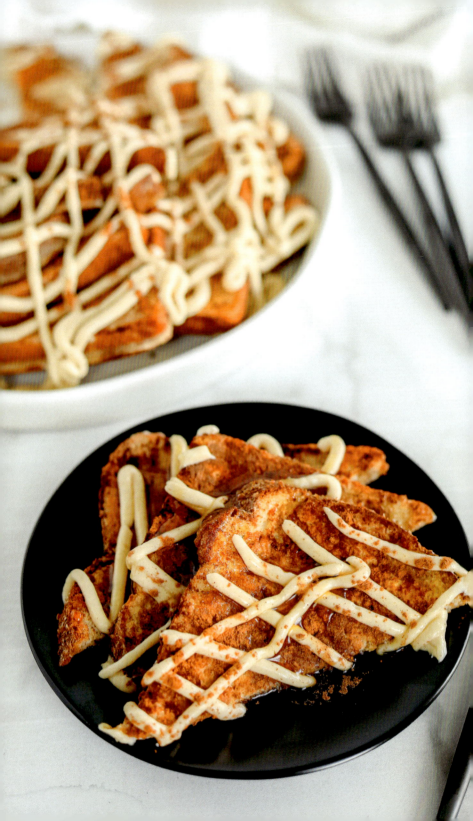

CINNAMON ROLL FRENCH TOAST

Makes 4 servings
300 calories / 11F / 35C / 21P / per serving

¼ cup fat-free milk
1 serving CSE Cinnamon Roll Protein Powder
2 large eggs
½ cup liquid egg whites
8 slices thin-sliced wheat bread (70-80
calories each) Cinnamon, to taste

Cream Cheese Glaze:
¼ cup (2 oz.) organic cream cheese
1 ½ Tbs. pure maple syrup
8g CSE Cinnamon Roll Protein Powder
1 Tbs. fat-free milk

Topping:
Walden Farms Pancake Syrup, optional

1. Make the Cream Cheese Glaze first by adding the cream cheese to a mixing bowl. Beat on high until smooth. Add the pure maple syrup, protein powder and milk. Mix together until well incorporated and smooth. Weigh the glaze and divide the total weight by 4 to get the amount needed to fill one serving. Set aside or store in the fridge until ready to use.

2. Heat griddle to medium heat.

3. Add the milk and the protein powder to a mixing bowl. Whisk together until smooth. Add the eggs and egg whites. Beat together until well combined.

4. Spray the griddle with cooking spray. Dip each slice of the bread into the mixture and then add to the griddle. Sprinkle cinnamon over the top of each slice of bread. Flip and cook to your liking on the other side.

5. Enjoy one serving (2 slices) of the Cinnamon Roll French Toast warm, topped with one serving of the Cream Cheese Glaze and syrup.

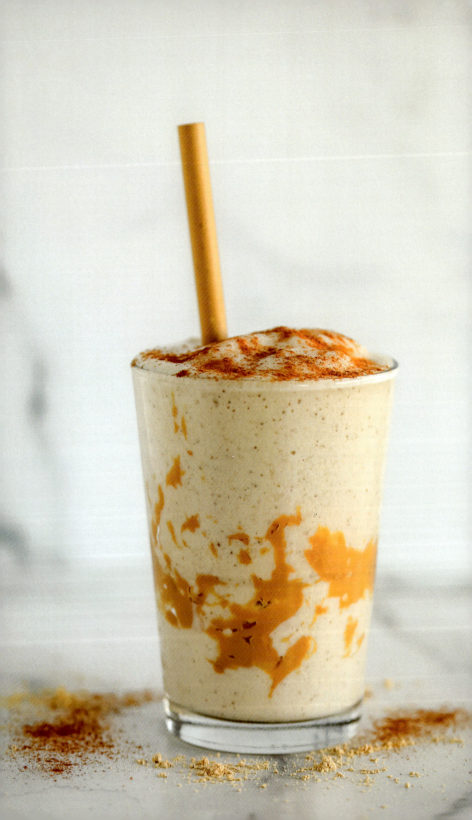

PB CINNA-BOMB SHAKE
Makes 1 serving
230 calories / 8F / 22C / 19P

---

1 cup unsweetened almond milk
¾ serving (25g) CSE Cinnamon Roll Protein Powder
60g frozen banana slices
2 tsp. (10g) OffBeat Sweet Classic Peanut Butter
   or natural peanut butter
½ tsp. chia seeds
6-8 (120g) ice cubes

1. Add all of the ingredients to a high-powered blender. Blend on high until smooth.

2. Pour into a cup. Enjoy!

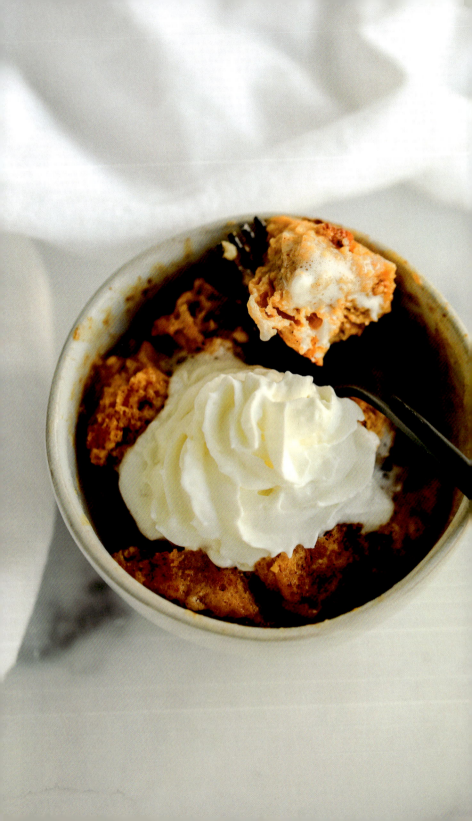

STICKY BUN MINUTE CAKE

Makes 1 serving
240 calories / 9F / 20C / 17.5P

---

1 Tbs. unsweetened almond milk
¼ tsp. baking powder
1 large egg
1 Tbs. pure maple syrup
½ serving (17g) CSE Cinnamon Roll Protein Powder
½ Tbs. OffBeat Cinnamon Bun Butter
   or natural almond butter
2 Tbs. spray whipping cream

1. Dissolve the baking powder into the almond milk in a small bowl. Beat in the egg, maple syrup and protein powder until well combined.

2. Spray a microwave safe bowl with cooking spray. Pour the mixture into the bowl, then fold in the OffBeat Butter. Place the bowl in the microwave and cook for 60-90 seconds. Enjoy warm topped with whipping cream.

COCONUT CREAM

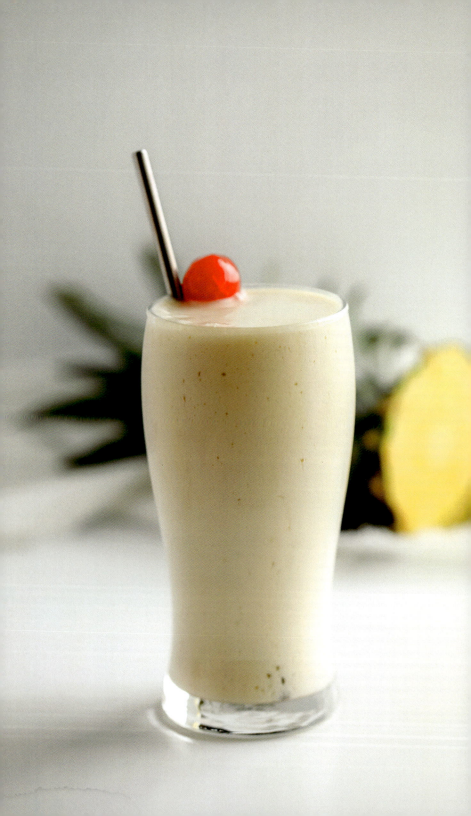

PINA COLADA SMOOTHIE

Makes 1 serving
250 calories / 8F / 23C / 21P

½ cup unsweetened almond milk
½ cup lite canned coconut milk
1 serving CSE Coconut Cream Protein Powder
125g fresh or frozen pineapple
6-8 (120g) ice cubes

1. Add all of the ingredients to a high-powered blender. Blend until smooth.

2. Pour into a cup. Enjoy!

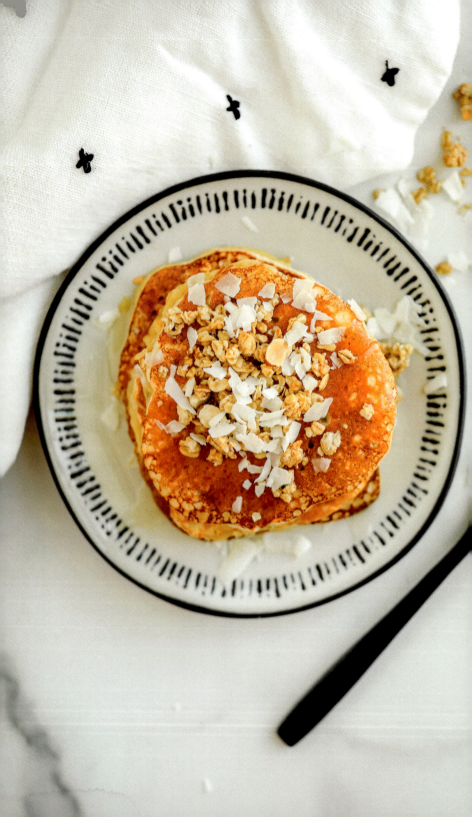

ISLAND COCONUT CRUNCH PANCAKES

Makes 1 serving
345 calories / 12F / 34C / 25.5P

¾ serving (25g) CSE Coconut Cream Protein Powder
2 Tbs. coconut flour
½ Tbs. unsweetened shredded coconut
¼ tsp. baking powder
Dash of sea salt
50g mashed bananas
1 large egg
3 Tbs. water
15g Nature's Path Coconut & Cashew Butter Granola

1. Heat griddle to medium heat.

2. Add the protein powder, coconut flour, shredded coconut, baking powder and sea salt to a small bowl. Mix until combined.

3. In a separate small bowl add the mashed banana, egg and water. Mix until combined. Add the wet ingredients to the dry ingredients and whisk together until well combined. Fold in the granola.

4. Using a ¼ measuring cup, scoop the batter onto the greased griddle. Once browned on one side, flip and cook on the other side. These brown quickly, so watch carefully. Enjoy as is or top with syrup or honey (not included in macros).

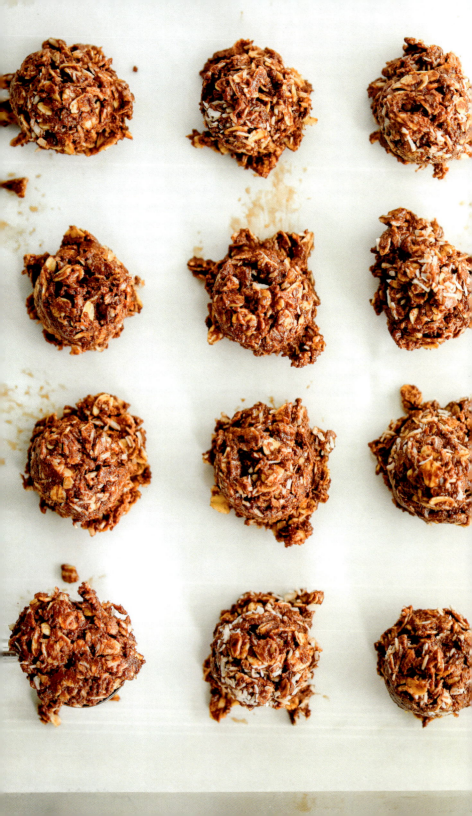

NO-BAKE MIDNIGHT COCONUT COOKIES

Makes 12 cookies
150 calories / 10F / 14C / 4P

¼ cup coconut oil
¼ cup coconut sugar
1 Tbs. raw honey
2 Tbs. unsweetened almond milk
2 Tbs. cocoa powder
⅓ cup OffBeat Midnight Almond Coconut Butter
   or natural almond butter
¼ cup unsweetened shredded coconut
1 cup old-fashioned rolled oats
1 serving CSE Coconut Cream Protein Powder

1. Add the coconut oil, coconut sugar, honey, almond milk and cocoa powder to a pot. Melt the ingredients down over medium/high heat. Whisk constantly until it starts to bubble. Turn heat off.

2. Stir in the nut butter, unsweetened shredded coconut and rolled oats. Add the protein powder last. Mix until well combined.

3. Using a small cookie scoop, scoop rounded cookies onto a baking sheet lined with parchment paper. Let cool and enjoy!

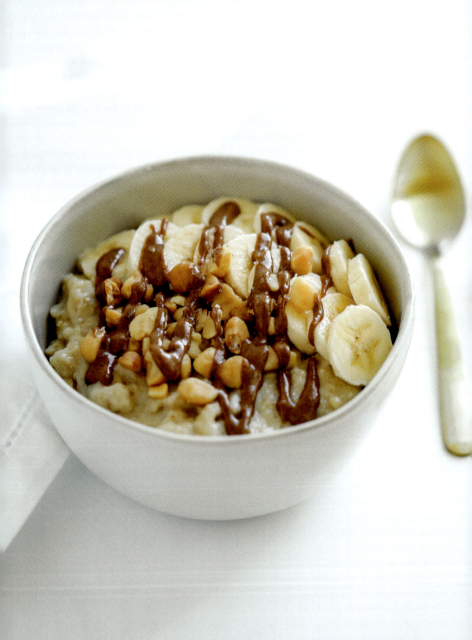

CHOCOLATE COCONUT MACADAMIA OATMEAL

Makes 1 serving
340 calories / 11.5F / 34C / 25.5P

⅓ cup old-fashioned rolled oats
½ cup water
3 Tbs. (46g) liquid egg whites
¾ serving (25g) CSE Coconut Cream Protein Powder
40g sliced bananas
8g chopped macadamia nuts
8g OffBeat Midnight Almond Coconut Butter
  or dark chocolate chips
Dash sea salt

1. Add the rolled oats, water and egg whites to a bowl. Microwave on high for 1.5 minutes or cook in a pot over medium heat for 5 minutes, stirring occasionally.

2. Remove from heat and stir. Let cool for a couple minutes. Add the protein powder and mix until well combined. Top with sliced bananas, macadamia nuts, OffBeat Butter/chocolate chips and sea salt. Enjoy!

* To make the oatmeal extra chocolatey, add a dash of cocoa powder when you add the protein powder and stir until well combined.

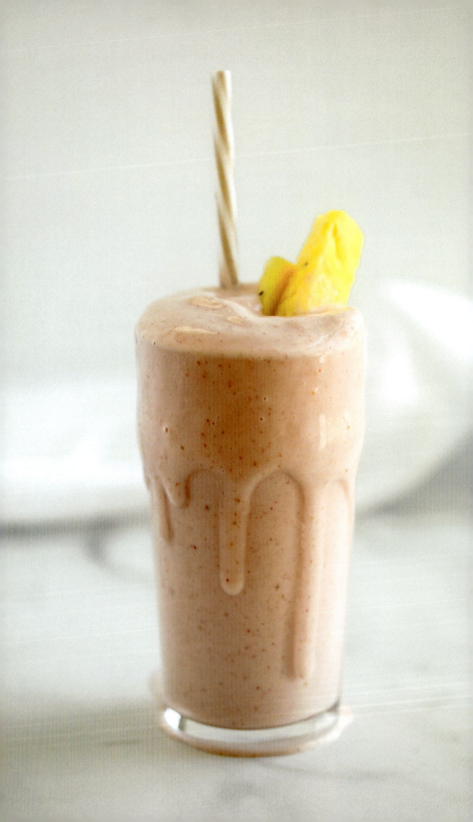

PEACHY COCONUT COLADA
(Post-Workout)
Makes 1 serving
230 calories / 2.5F / 21C / 32P

---

1 cup unsweetened almond or coconut milk
1 ½ servings (49g) CSE Coconut Cream
   or Peaches & Cream Protein Powder
100g fresh or frozen peaches
25g fresh or frozen pineapple
6-8 (100g) ice cubes

1. Add all of the ingredients to a high-powered blender. Blend until smooth.

2. Pour into a cup. Enjoy!

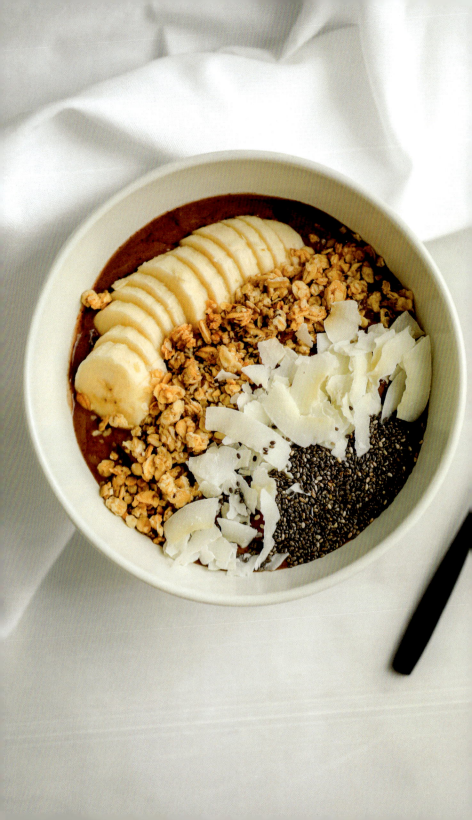

COCONUTTY ACAI BOWL

Makes 1 serving
340 calories / 12F / 36C / 23.5P

---

1 frozen Sambazon unsweetened acai pack
40g frozen banana slices
¼ cup unsweetened almond coconut milk
1 serving CSE Coconut Cream Protein Powder
80g ice cubes

Toppings:
20g banana slices
10g Nature's Path Coconut & Cashew Butter granola
5g unsweetened flaked coconut
¼ tsp. chia seeds
½ tsp. raw honey

1. Add the Acai to a high-powered blender; pulse until broken up. Add the frozen banana, almond coconut milk, protein powder and ice cubes. Pulse until broken up and smooth.

2. Pour into a bowl and top with banana slices, granola, coconut, chia seeds and honey. Enjoy!

EGGNOG

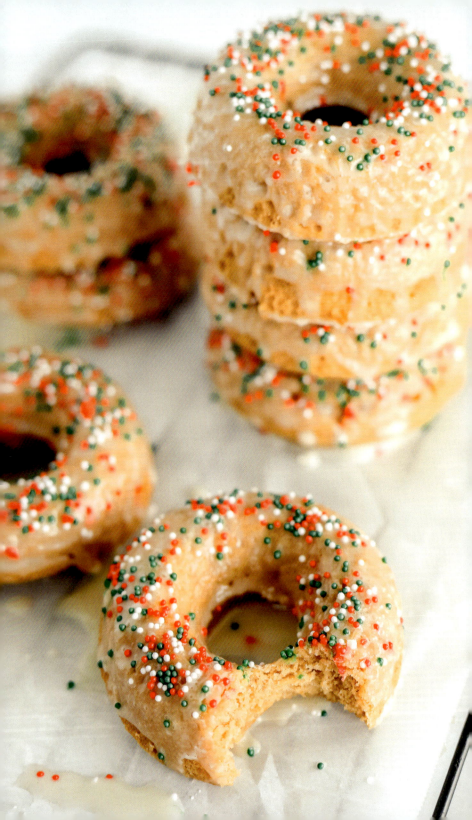

EGGNOG DONUTS

Makes 10 servings
160 calories / 4F / 28C / 4P / per serving

---

1 cup whole wheat pastry flour
1 serving CSE Eggnog Protein Powder
⅓ cup coconut sugar
¾ tsp. baking powder
¼ tsp. sea salt
¼ tsp. cinnamon
¼ tsp. nutmeg
½ cup unsweetened almond milk
1 large egg
½ tsp. vanilla extract
2 Tbs. coconut oil
Eggnog Icing:
1 cup powdered sugar
2 Tbs. almond milk eggnog
Sprinkles, optional

1. Preheat the oven to 425 degrees.

2. Add the flour, protein powder, coconut sugar, baking powder, sea salt, cinnamon and nutmeg to a large bowl. Whisk until combined. Set aside.

3. In a separate bowl, beat the almond milk, egg and vanilla extract. Add the wet ingredients to the dry ingredients and mix until just combined.

4. Melt the coconut oil and lightly whisk into the batter.

5. Spray donut molds with cooking spray. Fill the donut molds ¾ full. Bake for 6 minutes. Let cool a couple minutes, then transfer to a cooking rack.

6. Add the powdered sugar and almond milk eggnog to a bowl and beat until smooth. Dip each donut into the icing and return to the cooling rack. Let dry for a couple minutes, then dip each donut a second time. Top immediately with Christmas sprinkles. Enjoy!

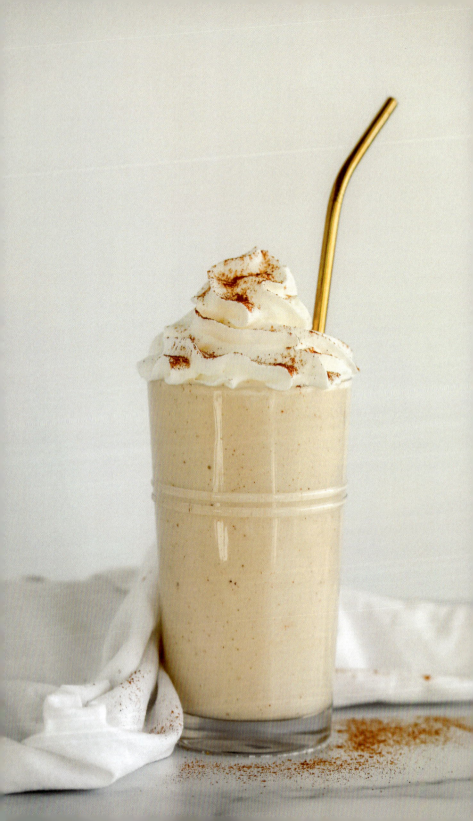

EGGNOG MILKSHAKE

Makes 1 serving
240 calories / 7F / 16C / 22P / per serving

---

1 cup unsweetened vanilla almond milk
1 serving CSE Eggnog Protein Powder
½ Tbs. OffBeat Gingerbread Cookie Butter
   or natural almond butter
30g frozen banana slices
 6-8 (120g) ice cubes
Toppings:
2 Tbs. spray whipping cream
Cinnamon, for garnish

1. Add all of the ingredients to a high-powered blender. Blend on high until smooth.

2. Pour into a cup. Enjoy!

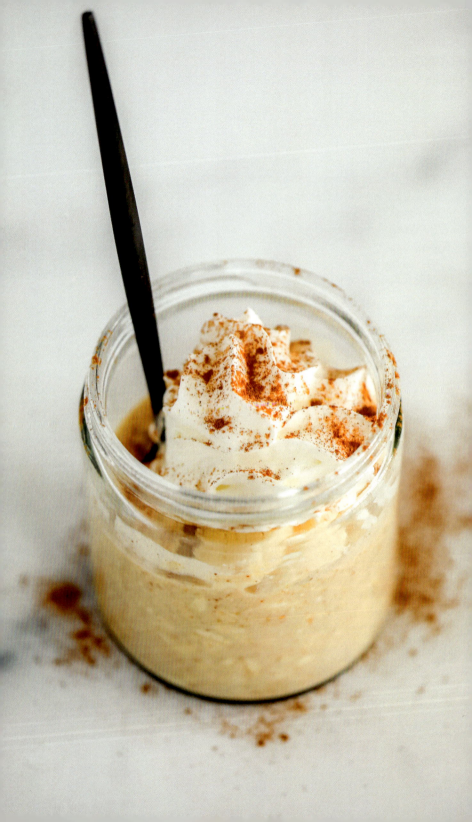

CHRISTMAS SPICED OVERNIGHT OATS

Makes 1 serving
355 calories / 11F / 44C / 22P

⅓ cup old-fashioned rolled oats
⅔ cup almond milk eggnog
¾ (24g) serving CSE Eggnog Protein Powder
1 Tbs. OffBeat Gingerbread Cookie Butter
Toppings:
20g banana slices
2 Tbs. spray whipped cream
Cinnamon, for garnish

1. Add all of the ingredients to a bowl or a jar and mix well. Cover and refrigerate overnight.

2. Top with banana slices, spray whipped cream and cinnamon. Enjoy cold.

*Stays good in the fridge up to 5-7 days

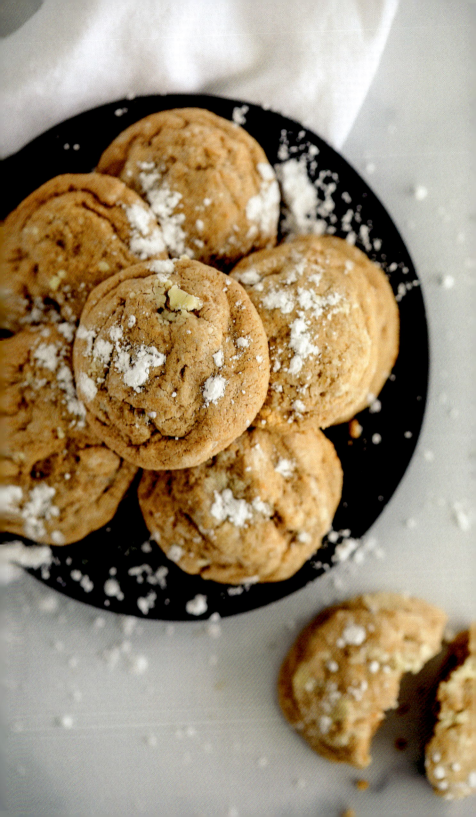

EGGNOG MELTAWAYS

Makes 12 servings
130 calories / 8F / 12C / 3P / per serving

¾ cup oat flour
¼ cup whole wheat pastry flour
3 Tbs. coconut sugar
½ tsp. cinnamon
½ tsp. baking soda
Dash sea salt
Dash nutmeg
½ cup grass-fed butter
1 serving CSE Eggnog Protein Powder
½ tsp. vanilla extract
2 Tbs. almond milk eggnog
 ¼ cup powdered sugar, for rolling

1. Add the flours, coconut sugar, cinnamon, baking soda, sea salt and nutmeg to a large bowl. Stir until combined. Set aside.

2. Add the softened butter and protein powder to a bowl. Beat until smooth. Beat in the almond milk and vanilla. Add the wet ingredients to the dry ingredients and mix until well combined.

3. Scrape down the sides of the bowl into the center. Cover and store in the fridge for 30-60 minutes.

4. Preheat the oven to 350. Using a small cookie scoop, scoop into balls. Roll each dough ball in powdered sugar and place on a baking sheet lined with parchment paper.

5. Bake for 6 minutes. Let cool and enjoy!

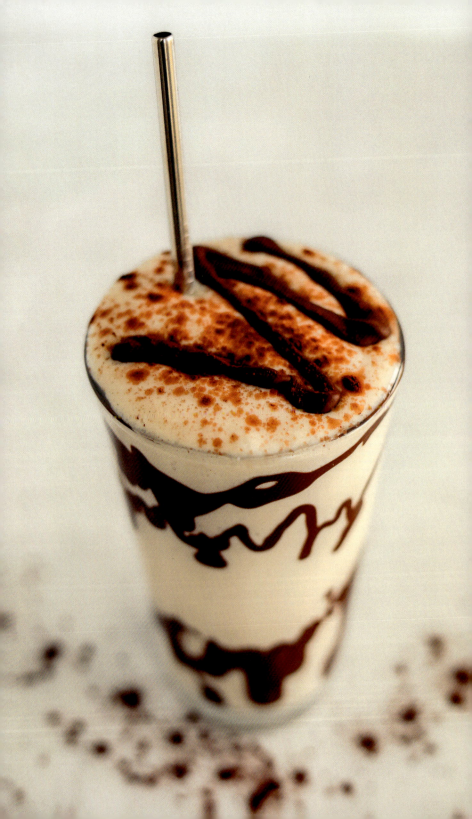

CHOCOLATE SWIRLED FROZEN EGGNOG

Makes 1 serving
310 calories / 10.5F / 31C / 23P / per serving

24g dark chocolate chips
1 cup unsweetened almond milk
1 serving CSE Eggnog Protein Powder
50g frozen banana slices
6-8 (120g) ice cubes
Topping:
Dash cocoa powder

1. Add the chocolate chips to a microwave safe bowl. Melt for 60-90 seconds, stirring every 30 seconds, until until smooth and melted. Drizzle the melted chocolate down the inside walls of a glass cup and set aside.

2. Add the rest of the ingredients to a high-powered blender. Blend on high until smooth.

3. Pour into the chocolate swirled cup. Sprinkle with cocoa powder and any remaining chocolate. Enjoy!

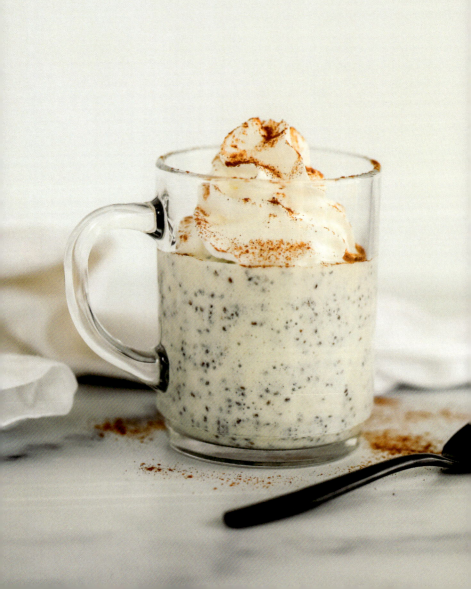

EGGNOG PUDDING

Makes 1 serving
250 calories / 9F / 19.5C / 22P / per serving

¼ cup almond milk eggnog
¼ cup plain Greek yogurt
½ (16g) serving CSE Eggnog Protein
Powder 2 Tbs. chia seeds
Toppings:
2 Tbs. spray whipping cream
Cinnamon, for garnish

1. Add all of the ingredients to a small bowl or jar. Mix until well com-bined. Store in the refrigerator overnight.

2. When ready to eat, top with whipping cream and cinnamon. Enjoy cold.

KEY LIME PIE

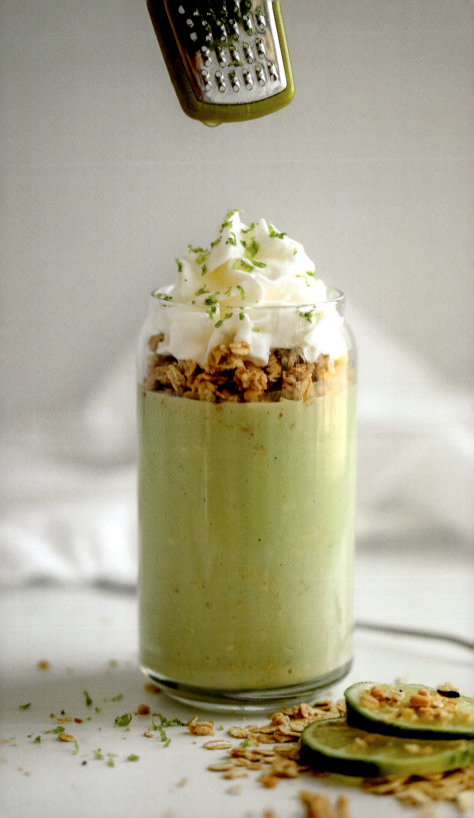

KEY LIME PIE OVERNIGHT OATS

Makes 1 serving
360 calories / 11F / 37C / 28.5P

---

2 Tbs. plain, fat-free Greek yogurt
25g avocado, sliced
½ lime, juice of
1 serving CSE Key Lime Pie Protein Powder
⅓ cup old-fashioned rolled oats
¾ cup unsweetened cashew or almond milk
Dash sea salt

Toppings:
1 Tbs. Key Lime Coconut Granola (see recipe below)
   or other granola of choice
1 Tbs. spray whipped cream
 ½ lime, zest of

1. Add the Greek yogurt, avocado and lime juice to a small mixing bowl. Using a hand mixer, beat all of the ingredients together until smooth.

2. Add the protein powder, rolled oats and milk. Stir together until well combined. Spoon into a jar or other container and let sit in the fridge overnight. When ready to eat, top with granola, spray whipped cream and lime zest. Enjoy!

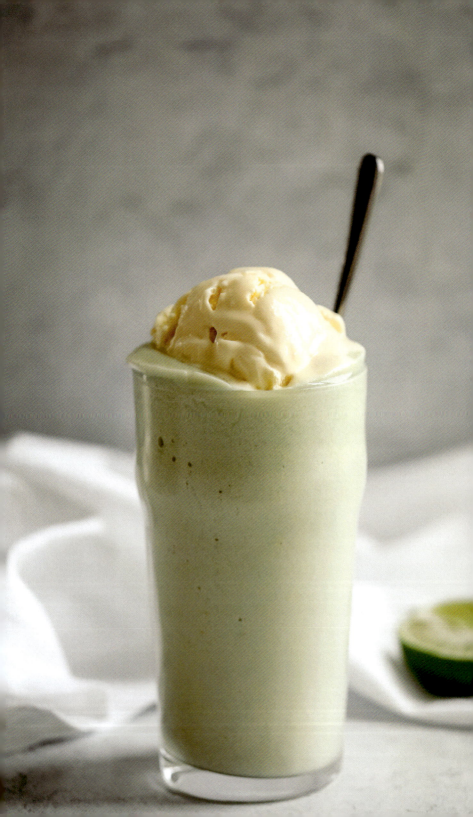

KEY LIME PIE MILKSHAKE

Makes 1 serving
350 calories / 11F / 30C / 28.5P

1 cup unsweetened vanilla almond milk
1 serving CSE Key Lime Pie Protein Powder
80g Key Lime (or vanilla) high-protein ice cream
10g OffBeat Lemon Coconut Bliss Butter
   or coconut butter
6-8 (120g) ice cubes

1. Add all of the ingredients to a high-powered blender. Blend until smooth.

2. Pour into a cup. Enjoy!

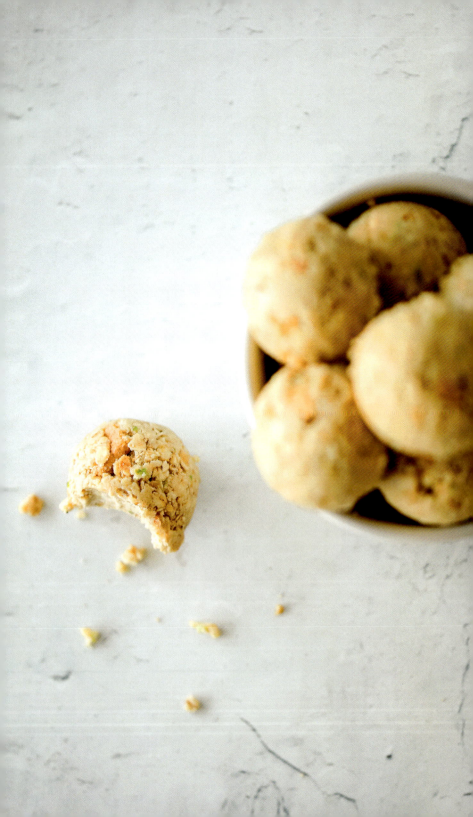

KEY LIME PIE BITES
Makes 28 bites
95 calories / 4.5F / 11C / 3P / per bite

---

1 cup OffBeat Aloha Butter
 or coconut butter
½ cup raw honey
2 servings CSE Key Lime Pie Protein Powder
1 cup old-fashioned rolled oats
Dash of sea salt
½ tsp. vanilla extract
Zest from 1 lime
½ cup graham cracker crumbs
 or Nature's Path Coconut & Cashew Butter Granola

1. Add all of the ingredients to a large mixing bowl. Mix until well combined.

2. Using a cookie scoop, scoop into balls and place in a container. Store in the fridge or freezer. Enjoy!

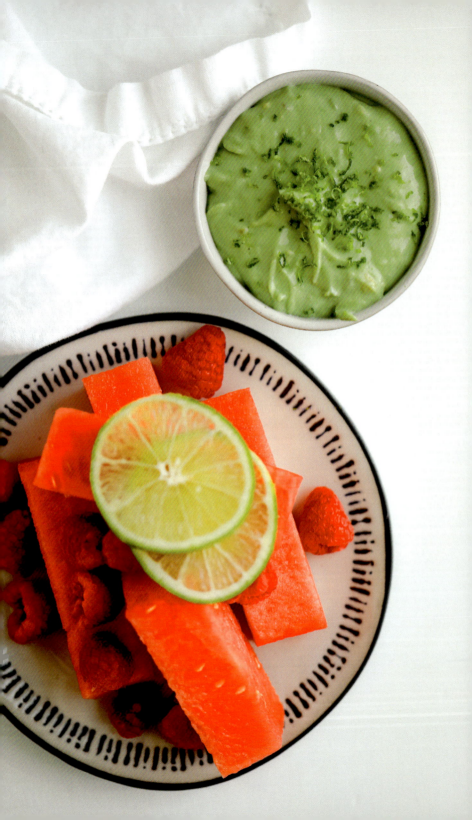

KEY LIME FRUIT DIP

Makes 1 serving
250 calories / 8F / 25C / 21P

¼ cup plain, fat-free Greek yogurt
35g avocado
¾ serving (24g) CSE Key Lime Pie Protein Powder
½ fresh lime, juice of
100g fresh watermelon
50g fresh berries

1. Add Greek yogurt, avocado, protein powder and lime juice to a small mixing bowl. Using a hand mixer, beat all of the ingredients together until smooth.

2. Use as a fruit dip or add the watermelon and the berries to the bowl and mix until combined. Enjoy!

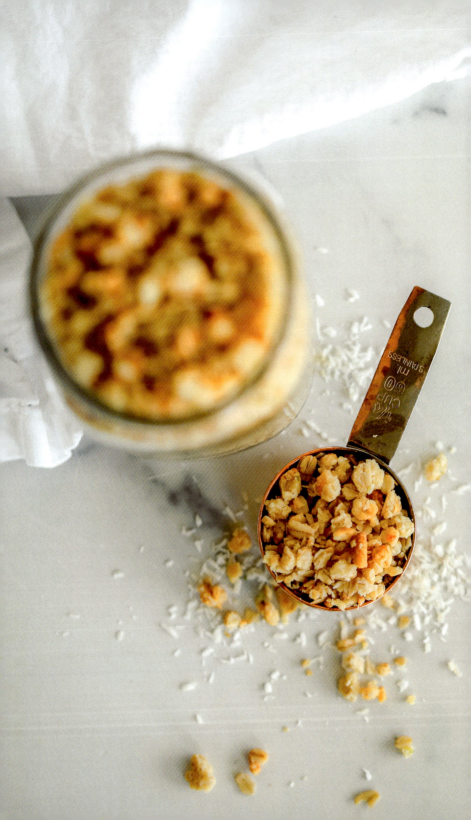

KEY LIME COCONUT GRANOLA

Makes 24 servings
130 calories / 7.5F / 13.5C / 2.5P / per serving

---

1 cup OffBeat Lemon Coconut Bliss Butter, Aloha Butter
  or softened coconut butter
½ cup raw honey
1 serving CSE Key Lime Pie Protein Powder
½ cup unsweetened shredded coconut
2 cups old-fashioned rolled oats
1 tsp. vanilla extract
½ tsp. sea salt
1 lime, zest of

1. Heat oven to 350 degrees.

2. Add all of the ingredients to a large mixing bowl. Mix until well combined.

3. Pour onto a baking sheet lined with parchment paper. Spread out into a single layer. Bake for 7-10 minutes, flipping halfway. Let cool, then place in a container and store in the fridge. Great on top of yogurt, ice cream, pancakes, with milk or as is.

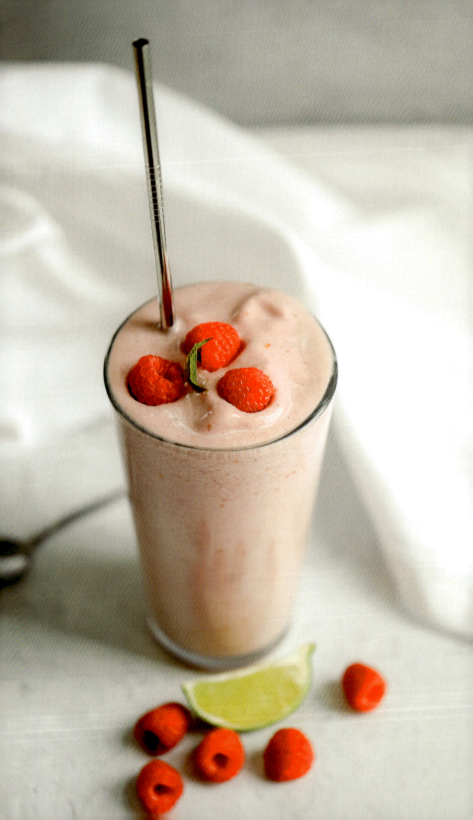

RASPBERRY KEY LIME SMOOTHIE (POST-WORKOUT)

Makes 1 serving
250 calories / 3F / 23C / 33P

---

1 cup unsweetened almond milk
1 ½ (49g) servings CSE Key Lime Pie Protein Powder
85g frozen raspberries
6-8 (120g) ice cubes

1. Add all of the ingredients to a high-powered blender. Blend until smooth.

2. Pour into a cup. Enjoy!

MAPLE DONUT

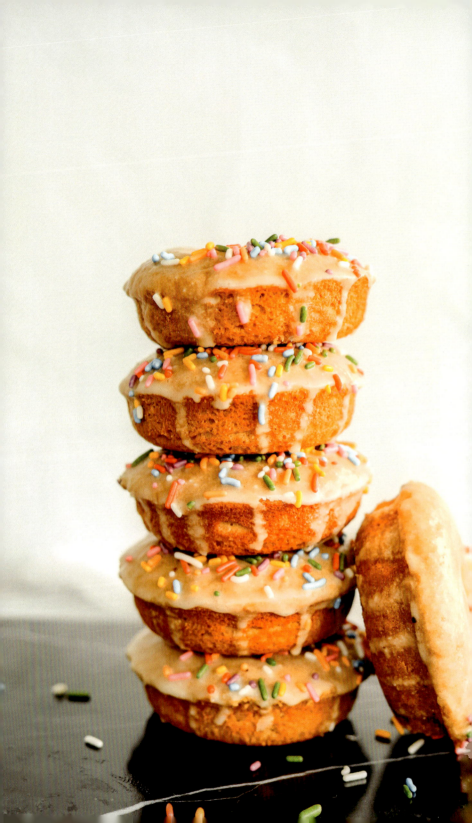

BAKED MAPLE DONUTS

Makes 12 servings
235 calories / 10F / 30.5C / 6P per donut

---

1 ¾ cup white whole wheat flour
1 serving CSE Maple Donut Protein Powder
½ Tbs. baking powder
½ tsp. baking soda
½ tsp. sea salt
2 large eggs
½ cup melted coconut oil
¼ cup unsweetened almond milk
¼ cup nonfat, plain Greek yogurt
¼ cup pure maple syrup
¼ cup coconut sugar
1 tsp. vanilla extract

Maple Glaze:
1 cup powdered sugar
2 Tbs. CSE Maple Donut Protein Powder
1-2 Tbs. unsweetened almond milk
½ tsp. vanilla extract
Sprinkles, optional

1. Heat the oven to 325 degrees. Grease donut pans with cooking spray.

2. Add the flour, protein powder, baking powder, baking soda and salt to a mixing bowl. Whisk together until well combined. Set aside.

3. In a separate mixing bowl, add the eggs, melted coconut oil, almond milk, yogurt, maple syrup, coconut sugar and vanilla extract. Beat together until smooth. Add the dry mixture to the bowl and mix on low speed until combined.

4. Transfer the batter to a large zip top bag. Cut a hole in the corner and pipe the batter into the donut pans filling each one ¾ full. Should make 12 donuts. Bake for 8 minutes. Let donuts cool in the pan for 5-10 minutes, then transfer to a cooling rack.

5. Add the powdered sugar, protein powder, milk and vanilla to a small mixing bowl. Beat together until smooth, adding more or less milk to reach desired consistency. Once the donuts are completely cooled, dip each donut in the glaze. Then dip again. Add sprinkles immediately before the glaze dries. Enjoy!

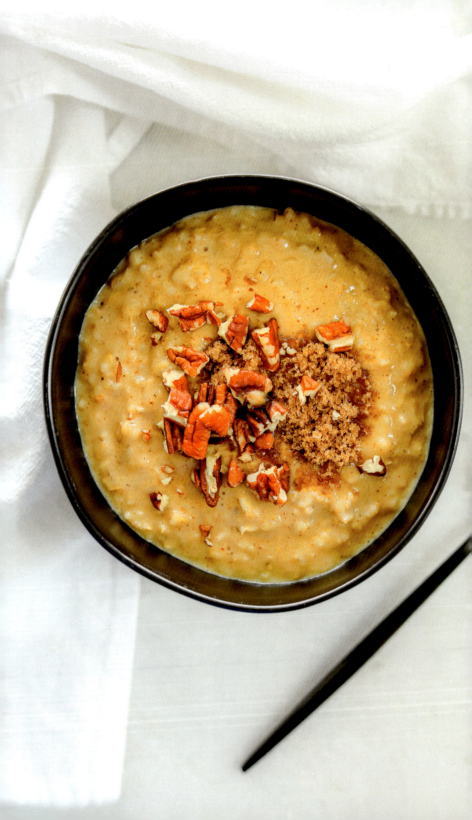

MAPLE & BROWN SUGAR OATMEAL

Makes 1 serving
340 calories / 12F / 31C / 26.5P

⅓ cup old-fashioned rolled oats
½ cup water
30g liquid egg whites
14g OffBeat Maple Donut Butter
  or natural almond butter
25g nonfat, plain Greek yogurt
Vanilla stevia drops, optional for sweetness
¾ serving (24g) CSE Maple Donut Protein Powder
1 Tbs. chopped pecans
1 tsp. coconut or brown sugar

1. Place the oats, water and egg whites in a microwave safe bowl. Whisk until the egg whites are well combined.

2. Microwave for 1-2 minutes.

3. Stir in the nut butter, yogurt and stevia until well combined. Add the protein powder and mix well. Top with chopped pecans and sugar. Enjoy!

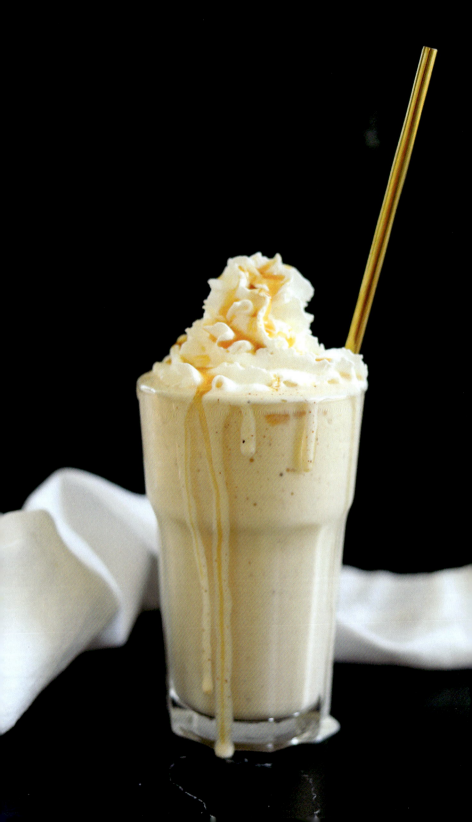

MAPLE DONUT MILKSHAKE

Makes 1 serving
340 calories / 10F / 35C / 27P

---

1 cup fat-free milk
1 serving CSE Maple Donut Protein Powder
20g OffBeat Maple Donut Butter
   or natural almond butter
40g frozen banana slices
1 tsp. pure maple syrup
Dash sea salt
6-8 (120g) ice cubes

1. Add all of the ingredients to a blender. Blend on high until smooth. Pour into a cup and enjoy!

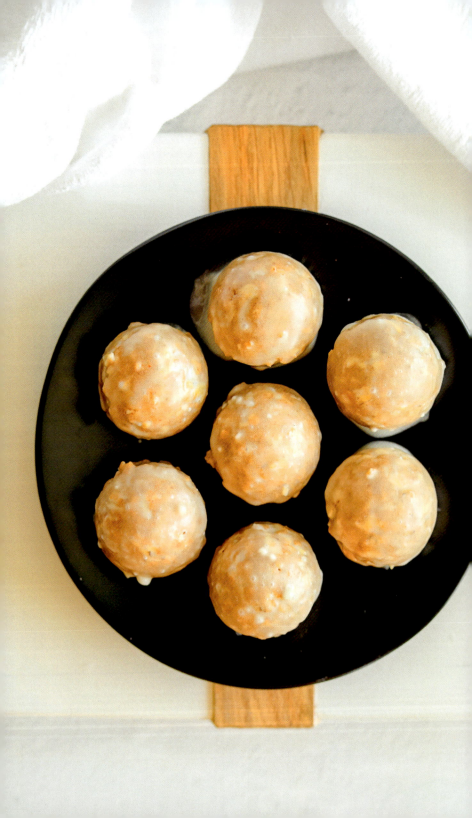

MAPLE DONUT HOLE POWER BITES

Makes 24 servings
110 calories / 5F / 14.5C / 3P per bite

1 cup OffBeat Maple Donut Butter
   or natural almond butter
½ cup raw honey
1 serving CSE Maple Donut Protein Powder
1 ½ cups old-fashioned rolled oats
Dash of sea salt
Dash of vanilla extract
Frosting:
½ cup powdered sugar
1 Tbs. liquid egg whites

1. Add the nut butter, honey, protein powder, oats, sea salt and vanilla to a mixing bowl. Mix until well combined. Set aside.

2. In a small bowl, whisk together the powdered sugar and egg whites. Set aside.

3. Using a cookie scoop, scoop the power bite mixture into balls and place on a baking sheet lined with parchment paper. Drizzle the frosting over the top of each one and store in the fridge until the frosting hardens. Move all the bites to a container, cover and store in the fridge or freezer.

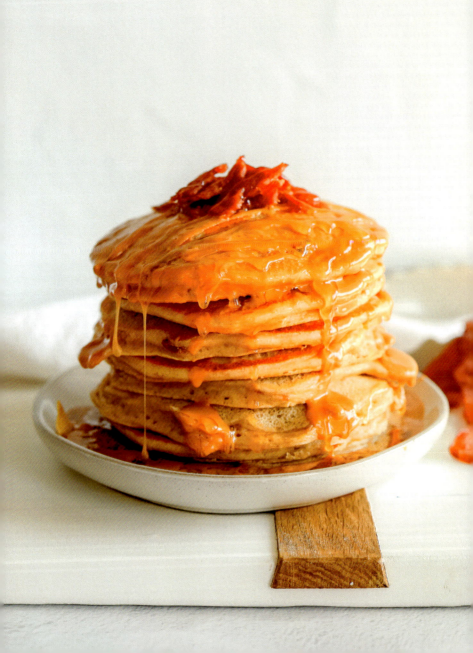

MAPLE BACON PANCAKES

Makes 4 servings
350 calories / 10.5F / 35C / 30P per serving

---

4 slices turkey bacon
2 cups CSE Vanilla Pancake & Waffle Mix
1 serving CSE Maple Donut Protein Powder
1 ½ cups water
Toppings Per Serving:
1 Tbs. OffBeat Sweet Classic Peanut Butter
  or natural peanut butter
Zero calorie syrup of choice

1. Heat a griddle to medium heat or 300 degrees. Cook the bacon on the griddle until crispy. Then chop into small pieces.

2. Add the CSE Pancake & Waffle Mix, protein powder and water to a mixing bowl. Whisk until smooth. Add the chopped turkey bacon and stir until well combined.

3. Using a ¼ measuring cup, pour the batter onto the greased griddle. Cook until golden brown on both sides.

4. Divide the pancakes into 4 equal servings and top each serving with peanut butter and syrup. Enjoy!

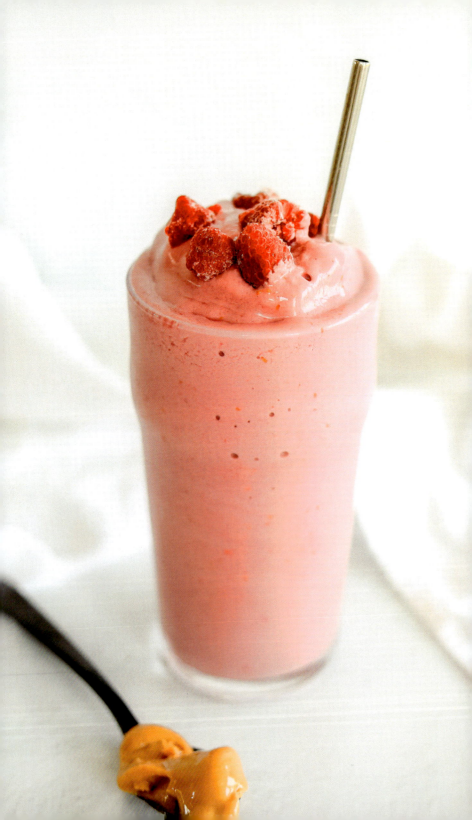

PB RASPBERRY MAPLE SHAKE

Makes 1 serving
240 calories / 7.5F / 23C / 21P

¾ cup unsweetened almond milk
¾ serving (24g) CSE Maple Donut Protein Powder
½ Tbs. OffBeat Sweet Classic Peanut Butter
   or natural peanut butter
¾ cup (120g) frozen raspberries
6-8 (120g) ice cubes
½ Tbs. powdered peanut butter

1. Add all of the ingredients to a high-powered blender. Blend on high until smooth.

2. Pour into a cup and top with powdered peanut butter. Enjoy!

MINT CHOCOLATE COOKIE

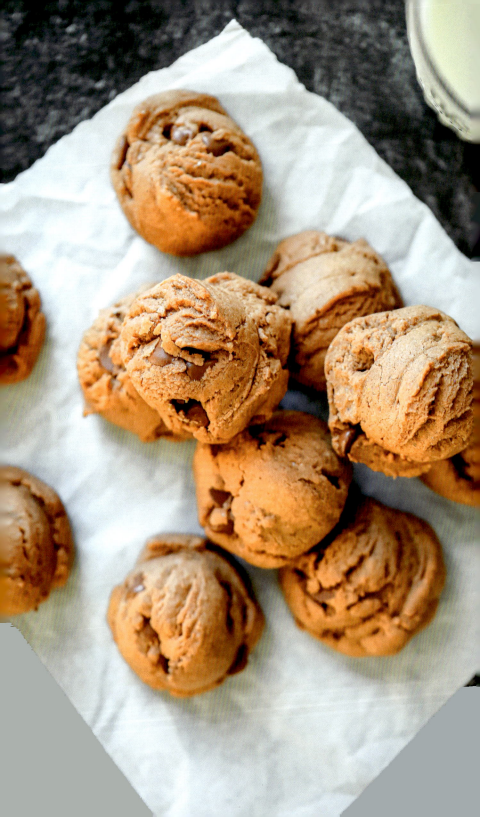

MINT CHOCOLATE CHIP COOKIES

Makes 16 cookies
150 calories / 9F / 14C / 4P / per serving

½ cup grass-fed butter
¼ cup OffBeat Mint Chocolate Chip Cookie Butter
1 serving CSE Mint Chocolate Cookie Protein Powder
⅓ cup organic cane sugar
1 large egg
1 tsp. vanilla extract
1 cup organic unbleached all-purpose flour
2 Tbs. cocoa powder
¼ tsp. sea salt
¼ tsp. baking soda
2 oz. dark chocolate chips

1. Preheat the oven to 350 degrees.

2. Add the butter, Mint Chocolate Chip Cookie Butter, Mint Chocolate Cookie Protein Powder and the sugar to a mixing bowl. Beat together until smooth. Add the egg and vanilla. Mix until combined.

3. In a separate bowl add the flour, cocoa powder, sea salt and baking soda and stir until combined. Add the wet ingredients to the dry ingredients and mix until just combined. Fold in the chocolate chips.

4. Using a cookie scoop, scoop the cookie dough onto a baking sheet lined with parchment paper. Bake for 8-10 minutes. Remove from the oven and allow to cool for a few minutes. Transfer to a cooling rack. Store leftover cookies in the fridge.

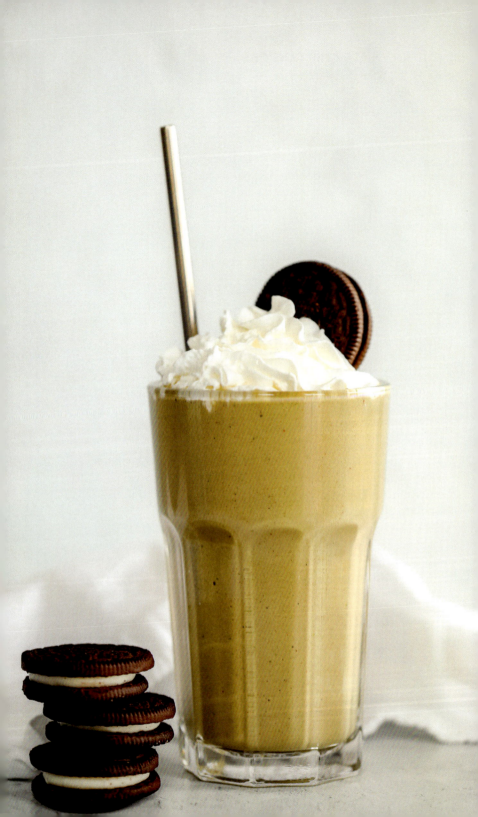

MINT COOKIES & CREAM SHAKE

Makes 1 serving
360 calories / 13.5F / 29C / 27P / per serving

---

1 cup unsweetened almond milk
¾ (24g) serving CSE Mint Chocolate Cookie Protein Powder
½ (7g) Tbs. OffBeat Mint Chocolate Chip Cookie Butter
¼ cup low-fat cottage cheese
1 Newman's Own Creme filled chocolate cookies
1 cup spinach
¼ tsp. xanthan gum
8-10 (150g) ice cubes

Topping:
2 Tbs. spray whipped cream
1 Newman's Own Creme filled chocolate
  cookies, crumbled

1. Add all of the ingredients to a high-powered blender. Blend until smooth and thick.

2. Pour into a cup and top with spray whipped cream and cookie crumbles. Enjoy with a spoon!

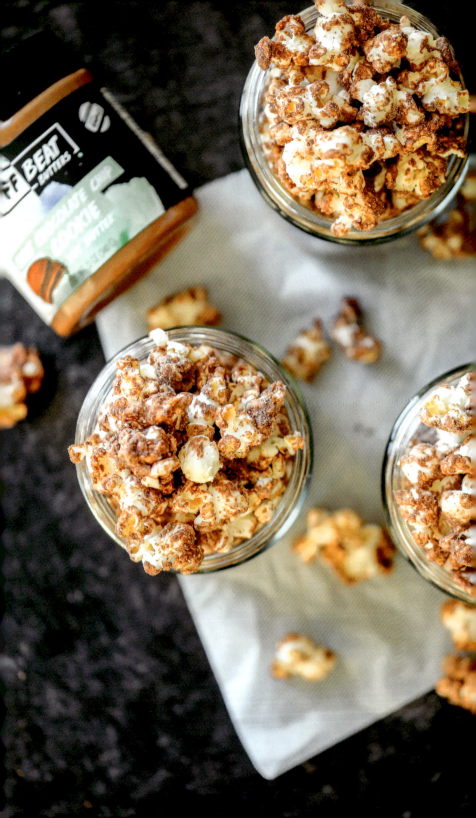

MINT CHOCOLATE POPCORN

Makes 8 servings / 1.25 oz. / per serving
170 calories / 10F / 15.5C / 5P / per serving

80g popcorn kernels
½ cup dark chocolate chips
¼ cup OffBeat Mint Chocolate Chip Cookie Butter
2 Tbs. grass-fed butter
1 tsp. vanilla extract
1 serving CSE Mint Chocolate Cookie Protein Powder

1. Air pop the kernels into a large bowl and set aside.

2. Add the chocolate chips, OffBeat Butter and butter to a small saucepan. Melt over low heat until smooth. Remove from heat and whisk in the vanilla extract.

3. Pour the melted chocolate mixture over the popcorn and mix gently until the popcorn is well coated. Immediately add the protein powder to the bowl and toss until the popcorn is well coated.

4. Divide into 8 servings and enjoy!

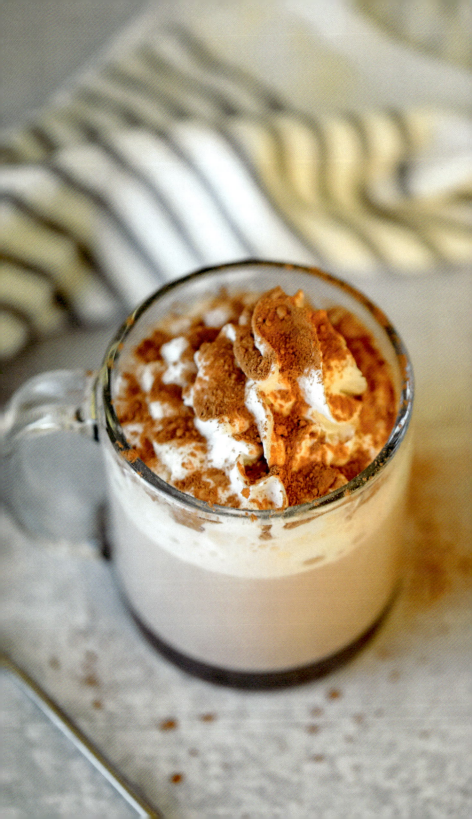

MINT HOT CHOCOLATE

Makes 1 serving

220 calories / 2F / 19C / 28P / per serving

---

1 cup fat-free milk
1 serving CSE Mint Chocolate Cookie Protein Powder
4 Tbs. spray whipped cream
Pinch of cocoa powder

1. Add the milk to a microwave safe mug. Heat in the microwave for 1 minute. Add the protein powder and mix with a milk frother until smooth. Heat for 15-30 more seconds, if needed.

2. Top with whipped cream and cocoa powder. Enjoy!

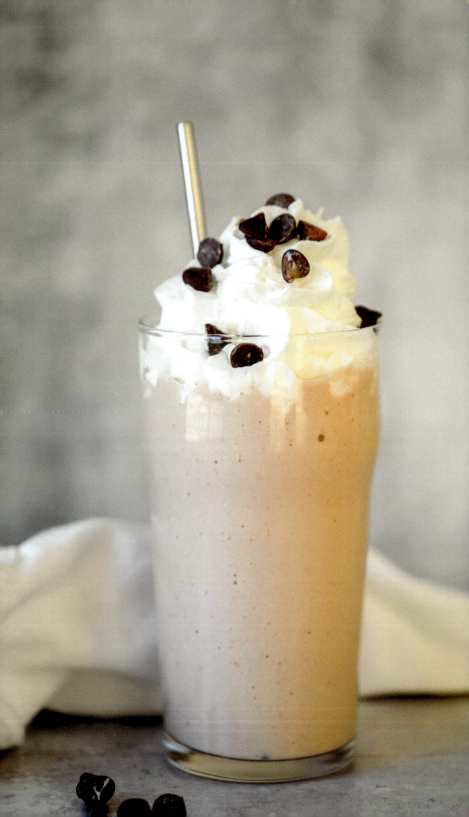

MINT CHOCOLATE COOKIE SHAKE

Makes 1 serving
240 calories / 9F / 16C / 23P / per serving

---

1 cup unsweetened almond milk
¾ serving (24g) CSE Mint Chocolate Cookie Protein Powder
½ Tbs. OffBeat Mint Chocolate Chip Cookie Butter
   or natural almond butter
1 Tbs. old-fashioned rolled oats
6-8 (120g) ice cubes
Toppings:
2 Tbs. spray whipped cream
5g dark chocolate chips

1. Add all of the ingredients to a high-powered blender and blend until smooth.

2. Pour into a cup. Top with whipped cream and dark chocolate chips. Enjoy with a spoon!

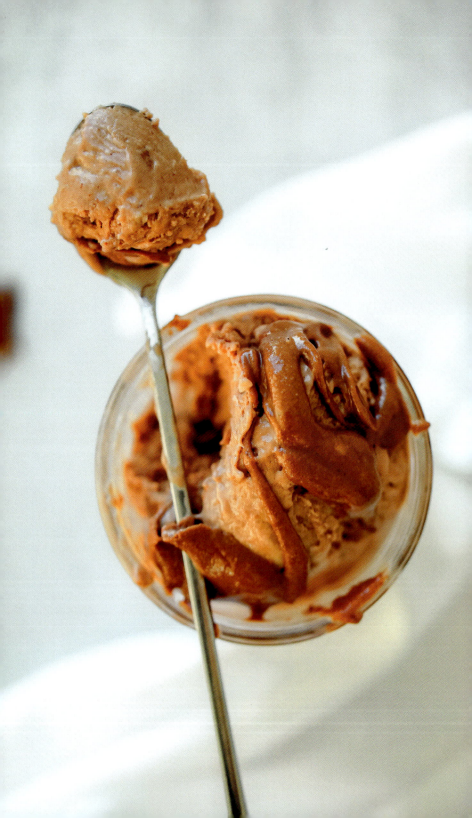

MINT CHOCOLATE ICE CREAM

Makes 4 servings
230 calories / 7.5F / 30C / 13P / per serving

400g frozen banana slices
2 servings CSE Mint Chocolate Cookie Protein Powder
¼ cup OffBeat Mint Chocolate Chip Cookie Butter
¼ cup unsweetened almond milk

1. Add all of the ingredients to a high-powered blender. Blend until smooth. Scrape down the sides in between blending until thick and smooth.

2. Scrape out into a loaf pan lined with parchment paper. Freeze for 2-3 hours. Use an ice cream scoop to scoop the ice cream into a bowl or cone. Divide into 4 equal servings. Top the ice cream with melted chocolate or extra Mint Chocolate Chip Cookie Butter. Enjoy!

PEACHES & CREAM

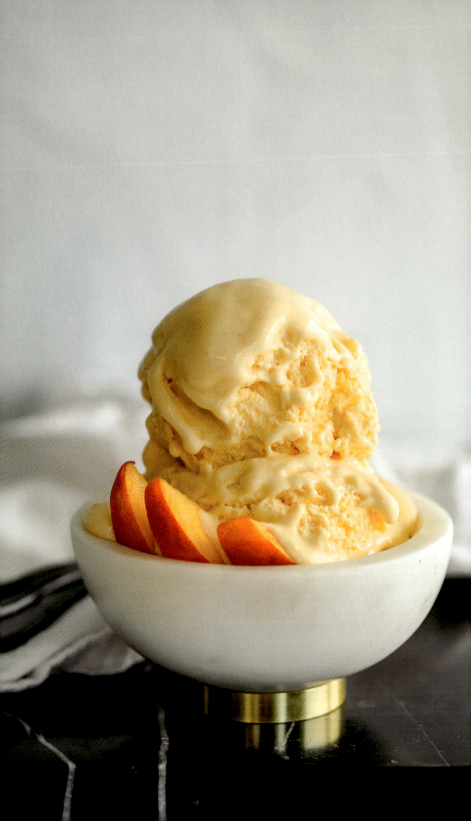

PEACH PROTEIN ICE CREAM

Makes 8 servings
255 calories / 15F / 19C / 11.5P per serving

---

2 cups (320g) peaches
2 Tbs. coconut sugar
1 ½ cups fat-free milk
1 ½ cups heavy cream
4 servings (132g) CSE Peaches & Cream Protein Powder
1 tsp. vanilla extract
Pinch sea salt

*You will need an ice cream maker for this recipe. Do all the preparation required of your ice cream maker beforehand.

1. Peel and chop the peaches then add them to a bowl. Sprinkle the coconut sugar over the top and stir until the peaches are well coated. Let sit for 15 minutes.

2. Once the juices from the peaches have released, add the peaches to a blender with ¼ cup of the milk. Blend until smooth. Pour back into the bowl.

3. Add the remaining milk, heavy cream, protein powder, vanilla extract and sea salt to the bowl. Whisk until smooth.

4. Start your ice cream maker and slowly add the ice cream mixture into the mixing bowl. Churn on low speed for 20 minutes or until the ice cream thickens up like soft serve. Enjoy as is or follow the next step for a more firm ice cream.

5. Place a piece of parchment paper into a 9x5 loaf pan, covering the bottom and sides of the pan. Scrape the ice cream into the pan and spread out evenly. Place in the freezer for 4-6 hours or overnight. Using an ice cream scoop, scoop into bowls and serve.

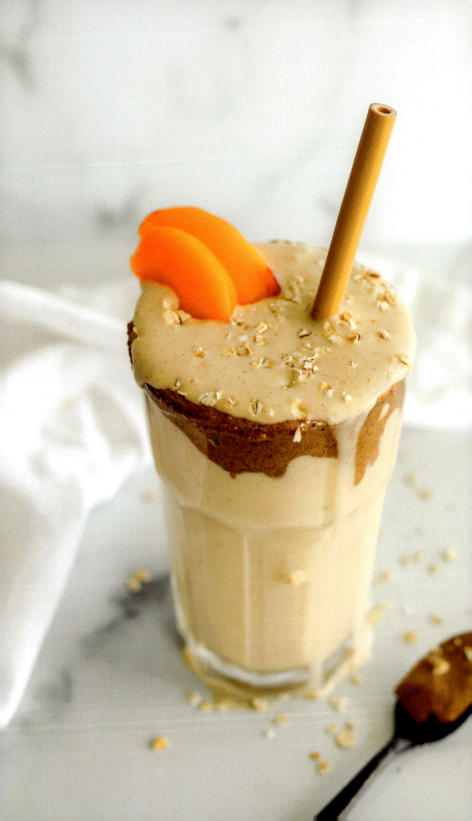

PEACH COBBLER SMOOTHIE

Makes 1 serving
335 calories / 10F / 32.5C / 29P

---

1 cup unsweetened almond milk
1 serving CSE Peaches & Cream Protein Powder
1 Tbs. OffBeat Cinnamon Bun Butter
  or natural almond butter
150g frozen peaches
2 Tbs. low-fat cottage cheese
2 Tbs. old-fashioned rolled oats
½ tsp. butter extract
Dash of cinnamon
Pinch of sea salt
6-8 (120g) ice cubes

1. Add all of the ingredients to a blender and blend on high until smooth. Pour into a cup and enjoy!

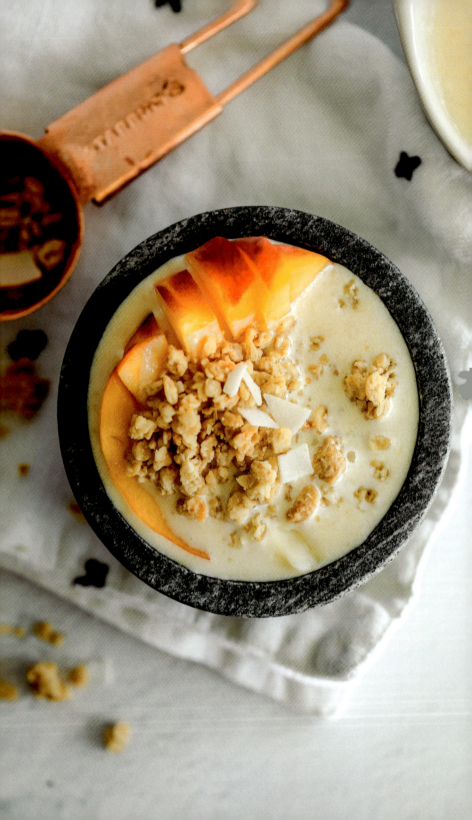

PEACHES & CREAM PARFAIT

Makes 1 serving
230 calories / 6F / 24C / 20P

½ cup nonfat, plain Greek yogurt
¼ serving (8.5g) CSE Peaches & Cream Protein Powder
Vanilla stevia drops, to taste
100g fresh sliced peaches
2 Tbs. Nature's Path Coconut & Cashew Butter Granola
2 Tbs. half & half

1. Add the yogurt, protein powder and stevia to a bowl. Mix until well combined. Top with peaches, granola and half & half. Enjoy!

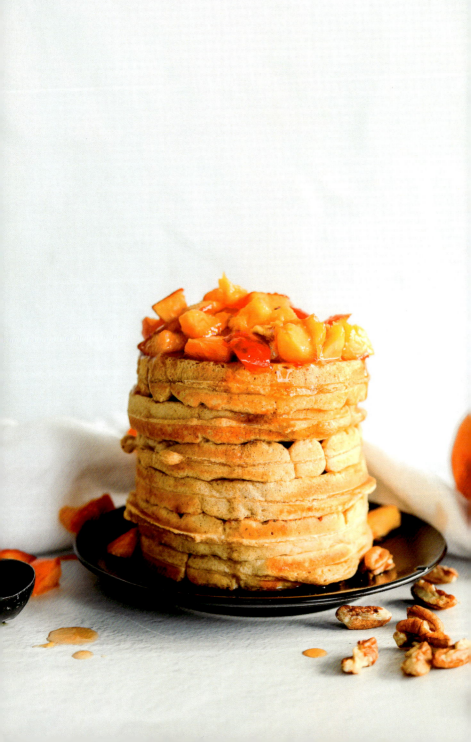

PEACH PECAN WAFFLES
Makes 4 servings
350 calories / 11F / 36C / 28.5P per serving

1 ½ cups CSE Vanilla Pancake & Waffle Mix
2 servings CSE Peaches & Cream Protein Powder
1 cup water
2 large eggs
⅓ cup nonfat, plain Greek yogurt
⅓ cup chopped pecans
1 Tbs. cinnamon
Toppings:
1 cup fresh peaches
1 Tbs. raw honey

1. Heat a waffle iron.

2. Combine the CSE Pancake & Waffle Mix, protein powder, water, eggs and Greek yogurt in a large bowl. Mix until well combined. Fold in the chopped pecans and cinnamon.

3. Pour into the waffle iron and cook until the outside is golden and crispy. Weigh the waffles and divide by four to get the amount needed to fill one serving.

4. While the waffles are cooking, add the peaches to a large, greased frying pan over low/medium heat. Stir until the peaches begin to soften. Drizzle the honey over the top and stir until the peaches are well coated. Remove from heat.

5. Top each serving of waffles with ¼ of the caramelized peaches and enjoy warm. Top with syrup if desired.

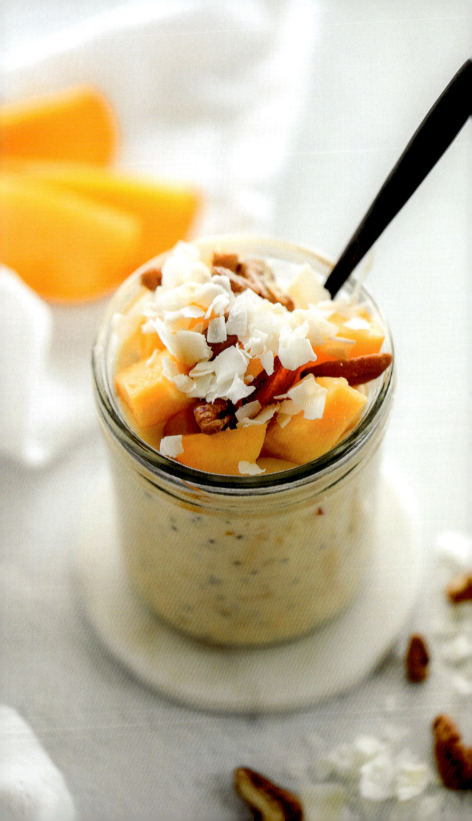

PEACH COCONUT PECAN OVERNIGHT OATS

Makes 1 serving
330 calories / 12F / 35C / 24P

⅓ cup old-fashioned rolled oats
½ cup coconut milk (from the carton)
¼ cup nonfat, plain Greek yogurt
¾ serving (24g) CSE Peaches & Cream Protein Powder
½ tsp. chia seeds
Vanilla stevia drops, to taste
Toppings:
50g fresh peaches
5g unsweetened flaked coconut
5g chopped pecans

1. Add the oats, coconut milk, Greek yogurt, protein powder, chia seeds and stevia to a bowl. Stir until well combined. Cover and refrigerate overnight.

2. When ready to eat, add all the toppings to the oatmeal and enjoy cold. *stays good in the fridge for 5-7 days.

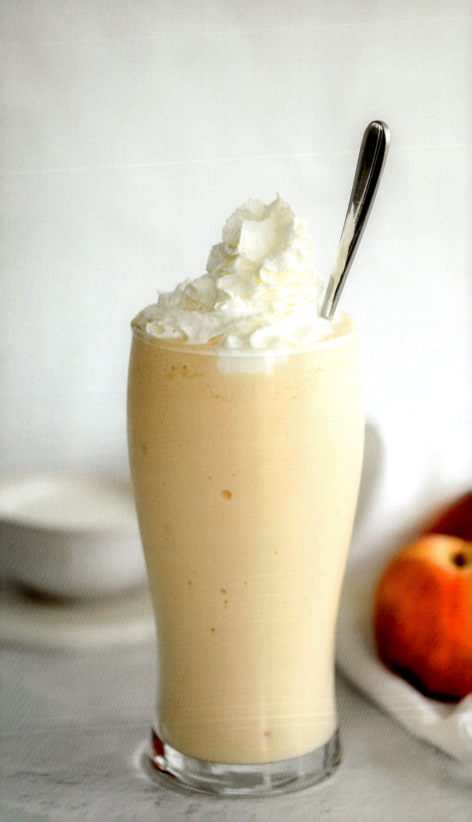

PEACHES & CREAM SHAKE

Makes 1 serving
350 calories / 12.5F / 30.5C / 28P

½ cup unsweetened almond milk
⅓ cup half & half
1 serving CSE Peaches & Cream Protein Powder
200g fresh or frozen peaches
2 Tbs. low-fat cottage cheese
Splash vanilla extract
6-8 (120g) ice cubes
Topping:
4 Tbs. (10g) spray whipped cream

1. Add all of the ingredients to a blender and blend on high until smooth. Pour into a cup and enjoy!

PUMPKIN PIE

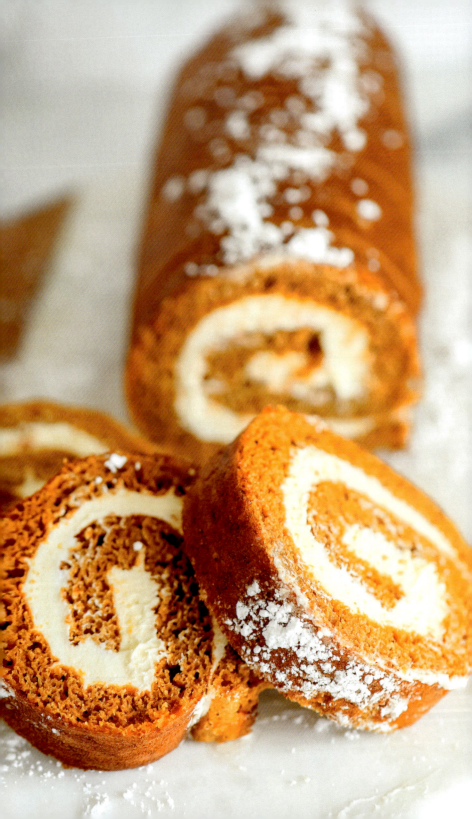

PUMPKIN ROLL
Makes 10 servings
320 calories / 13F / 43C / 8.5P / per serving

---

1 serving CSE Pumpkin Pie Protein Powder
½ cup whole wheat pastry flour
½ tsp. baking powder
½ tsp. baking soda
½ Tbs. pumpkin pie spice
¼ teaspoon salt
3 large eggs
1 tsp. vanilla extract
1 cup coconut sugar
⅔ cup canned pumpkin
¼ cup powdered sugar, optional for garnish
Cream Cheese Filling:
1 (8 ounce) Neufchâtel cream cheese (room temperature)
6 Tbs. grass-fed butter (room temperature)
1 serving CSE Simply Vanilla Protein Powder
3 Tbs. raw honey
1 tsp. vanilla extract

1. Preheat the oven to 375 degrees. Place parchment paper into a 10x15" rimmed baking sheet leaving about an inch of the parchment paper hanging over the edges of all sides of the pan.

2. Add the protein powder, flour, baking powder, baking soda, pumpkin pie spice and salt to a large mixing bowl. Stir until well combined.

3. In a separate mixing bowl, add the eggs, vanilla extract and coconut sugar. Whisk together until just combined, then whisk in the pumpkin until smooth. Add the wet ingredients to the dry and mix until just combined.

4. Pour the cake batter into the prepared pan. Spread the batter out evenly with a rubber spatula, coating the entire pan. Bake for 10-12 minutes.

5. Remove from the oven and then holding the sides of the parchment paper, remove the cake from the pan and set on the counter. Slowly roll the cake, leav-ing the parchment paper on and place on a cooling rack. Let cool completely.

6. Make the filling by adding the cream cheese and the butter to a small mixing bowl. Beat together until smooth. Add the protein powder and beat until smooth. Add the honey and the vanilla and beat until smooth.

7. Unroll the cake and spread the cream cheese filling evenly over the entire cake. Gently roll the cake back up with the cream cheese filling now on the in-side. This time, carefully remove the parchment paper from the cake as you roll it up. Wrap the pumpkin roll in plastic wrap and store in the fridge until ready to serve. Top with powdered sugar and cut into 10 even slices. Enjoy!

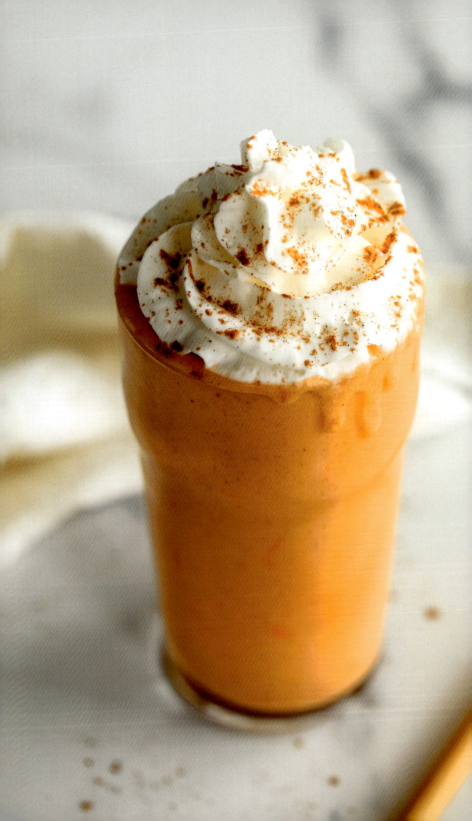

PUMPKIN PIE SHAKE

Makes 1 serving
345 calories / 11F / 35.5C / 26P

---

1 cup unsweetened almond milk
1 serving CSE Pumpkin Pie Protein Powder
¼ cup canned pumpkin
80g frozen banana slices
1 Tbs. OffBeat Cinnamon Bun Butter
  or natural almond butter
Dash pumpkin pie spice

Topping:
2 Tbs. spray whipped cream

1. Add all of the ingredients to a high-powered blender. Blend on high until smooth.

2. Pour into a cup. Top with whipped cream. Enjoy!

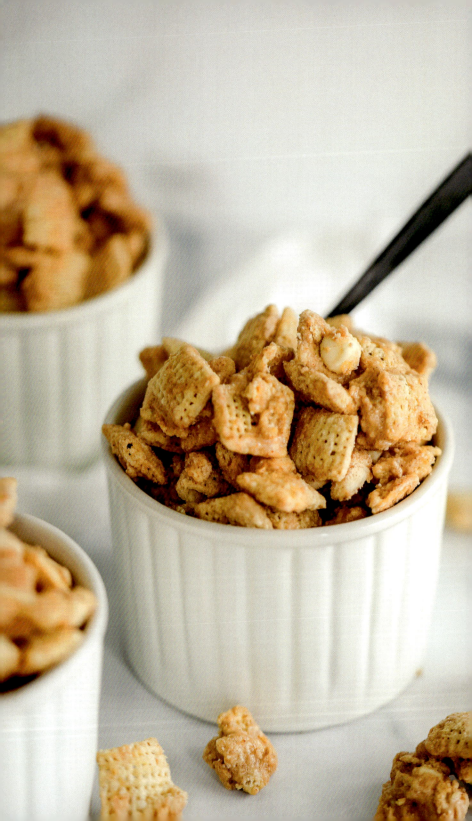

PUMPKIN PIE PUPPY CHOW

Makes 12 servings
310 calories / 15F / 38C / 8P / per serving

7 cups Chex Rice Cereal
1 cup graham cracker crumbs
1 cup white chocolate chips
¼ cup grass-fed butter
½ cup OffBeat Pumpkin Spice Butter
¼ cup raw honey
Pinch of sea salt
Dash of cinnamon
2 servings CSE Pumpkin Pie Protein Powder

1. Pour the cereal, graham cracker crumbs and ½ cup of the chocolate chips into a large bowl; set aside.

2. Add the butter to a small saucepan over low heat. Once melted, add the nut butter, honey, ½ cup white chocolate chips, sea salt and cinnamon. Stir constantly until completely melted. Remove from heat and let cool for a couple minutes. Stir in one serving of the protein powder.

3. Pour the hot mixture over the top of the dry mixture in the bowl. Stir until well coated. Sprinkle with another serving of protein powder. Stir and serve. One serving is approx 1 cup or 75 grams.

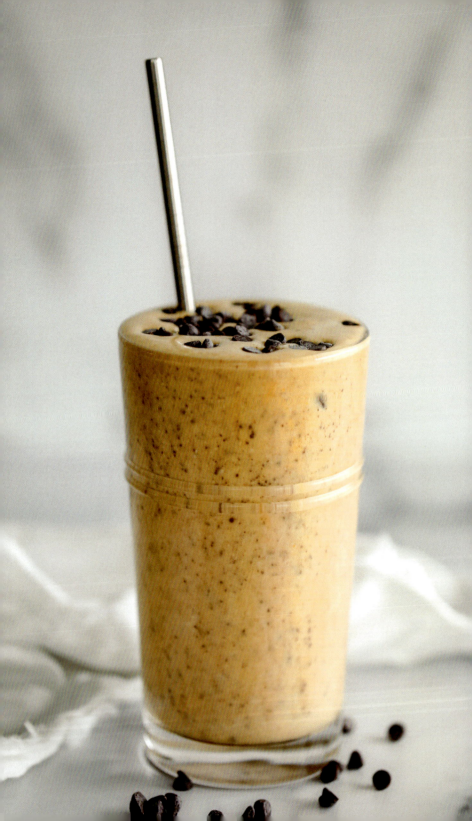

PUMPKIN CHOCOLATE SPECKLED SHAKE

Makes 1 serving
250 calories / 9F / 23.5C / 18.5P

---

1 cup unsweetened almond milk
¾ serving CSE Pumpkin Pie Protein Powder
2 Tbs. canned pumpkin
40g frozen banana slices
½ Tbs. (7g) OffBeat Pumpkin Spice or Cinnamon Bun Butter
   or natural almond butter
½ Tbs. (7g) mini chocolate chips
6-8 (120g) ice cubes

1. Add all of the ingredients to a high-powered blender. Blend until smooth.

2. Pour into a cup. Enjoy!

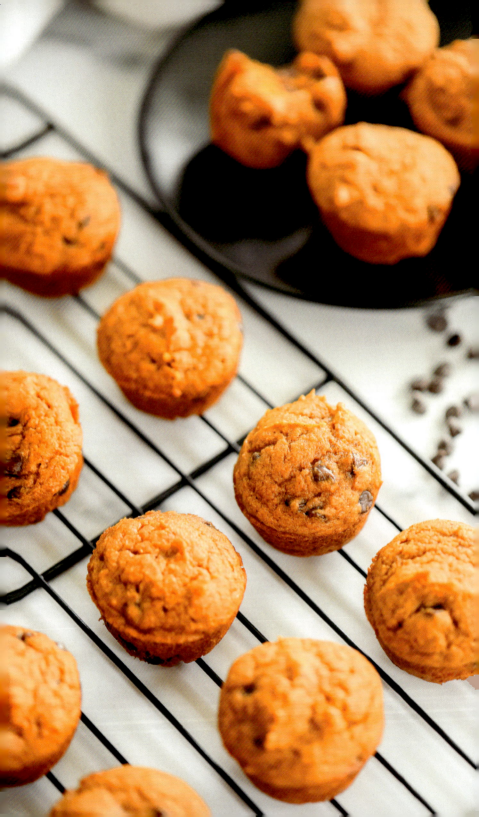

MINI PUMPKIN CHOCOLATE CHIP MUFFINS

Makes 46 mini muffins
40 calories / 1.5F / 5.5C / 1.5P / per muffin

1 serving CSE Pumpkin Pie Protein Powder
1 ½ cups Kodiak Cakes Pumpkin Flax Mix
1 tsp. Baking soda
1 tsp. Baking powder
½ tsp. Sea salt
½ tsp. Cinnamon
2 large eggs
1 cup canned pumpkin
1 tsp. Vanilla extract
½ cup coconut sugar
¼ cup nonfat, plain Greek yogurt
¼ cup melted butter
⅓ cup fat-free milk
½ cup mini chocolate chips

1. Preheat the oven to 350 degrees. Grease a mini muffin tin. No liners needed.

2. Add the protein powder, Kodiak Cakes Mix, baking soda, baking powder, sea salt and cinnamon to a large bowl. Stir until combined; set aside.

3. In a separate bowl, whisk the eggs, pumpkin, vanilla, coconut sugar, Greek yogurt, melted butter and milk together until well combined. Add the wet ingredients to the dry and whisk until just combined. Fold in the chocolate chips.

4. Spoon about 1 Tbs. of the batter into each muffin cup, filling about ¾ of the way full. Bake for 12 minutes. Let cool for a couple minutes. Transfer to a cooling rack.

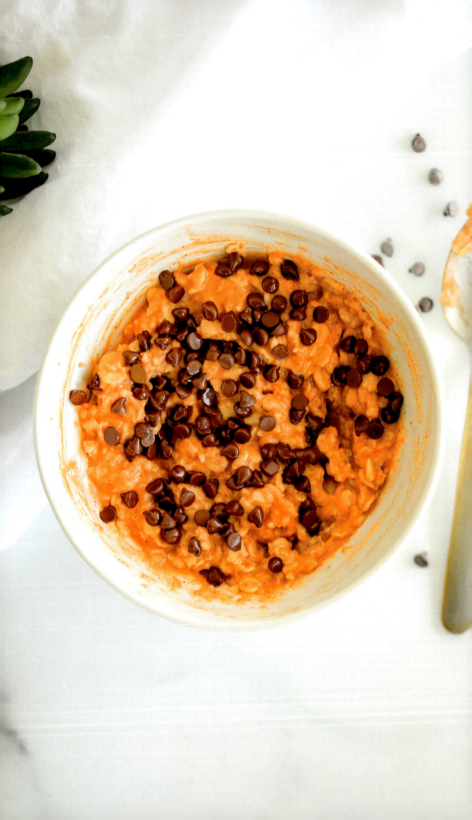

PUMPKIN CHOCOLATE CHIP COOKIE OATMEAL

Makes 1 serving

355 calories / 12F / 35C / 26.5P

⅓ cup old-fashioned rolled oats
½ cup water
3 Tbs. (46g) egg whites
1 Tbs. (14g) OffBeat Pumpkin Spice Butter
  or natural almond butter
¾ (24g) serving CSE Pumpkin Pie Protein Powder
Dash of sea salt
Vanilla stevia drops, optional to taste
Unsweetened almond milk, optional to taste
1 Tbs. (15g) mini chocolate chips

1. Add the oats, water and egg whites to a bowl. Microwave for 1.5 minutes or cook on the stovetop for 3-5 minutes.

2. Add the nut butter and stir until well combined. Let cool for a couple minutes. Stir in the protein powder, salt, stevia and a little almond milk if the oatmeal is too thick. Sprinkle the chocolate chips over the top. Enjoy!

S'MORES

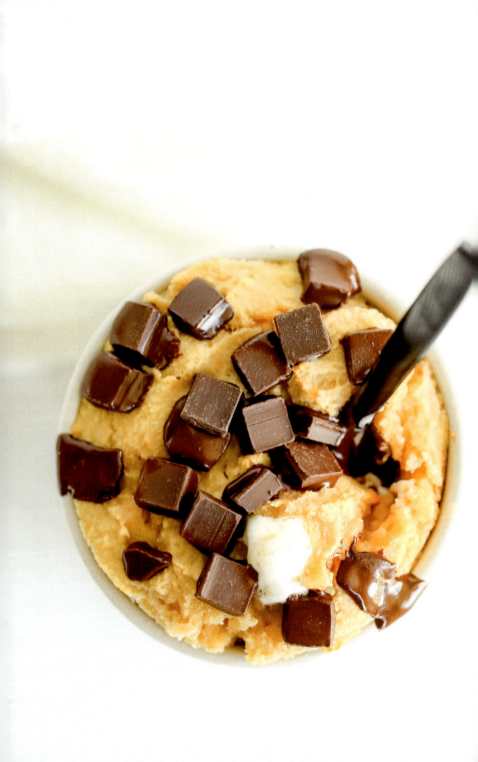

S'MORES BLONDIE
Makes 1 serving
350 calories / 11.5F / 34C / 25.5P

4-5 Tbs. unsweetened almond milk
1 large egg
¾ serving (24g) CSE S'mores Protein Powder
3 Tbs. coconut flour
½ tsp. baking powder
2 Smashmallow marshmallows
   (Cinnamon Churro, Toasted Vanilla or Cookie Dough)
Topping:
10g chocolate chips

1. Add the almond milk and egg to a bowl and whisk until smooth. Add the protein powder, coconut flour and baking powder. Stir until well combined.

2. Grease a small oven/microwave safe bowl or mug with cooking spray. Pour ½ of the mixture into the bowl/mug. Add the marshmallows and then cover them with the remaining mixture.

3. Microwave for 1-2 minutes on high or bake at 350 for 13-15 minutes. Should still look a little gooey, do not overcook. Top with chocolate chips and enjoy!

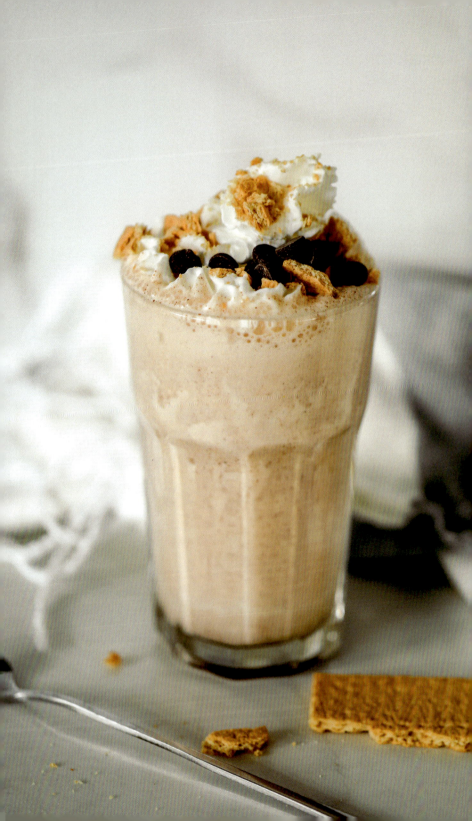

S'MORES PROTEIN SHAKE

Makes 1 serving
340 calories / 9F / 33C / 33P

1 cup unsweetened cashew milk
1 ½ (50g) servings CSE S'mores Protein Powder
¼ tsp. xanthan gum
40g frozen banana slices
150g ice cubes

Toppings:
½ sheet of graham crackers, crumbled
30 (15g) dark chocolate chips
2 Tbs. spray whipping cream

1. Add the cashew milk, S'mores Protein Powder, xanthan gum, banana slices and ice to a blender. Blend on high until thick and smooth. Pour into a large cup.

2. Top with crumbled graham crackers, chocolate chips and whipping cream. Enjoy with a spoon.

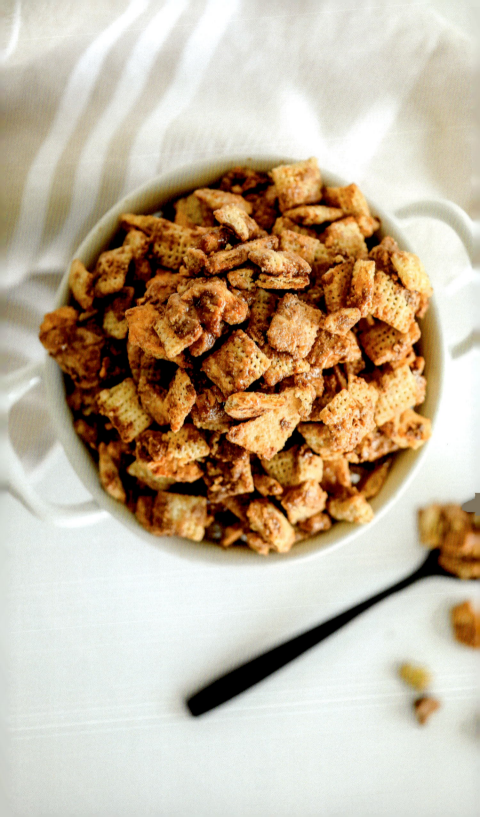

S'MORES PUPPY CHOW
Makes 12 servings
310 calories / 15F / 38C / 8P / per 80g serving

---

7 cups Rice Chex Cereal
5 graham cracker sheets (about 1 cup crumbled)
½ cup chocolate chips
¼ cup grass-fed butter
½ cup natural almond butter or peanut butter
¼ cup raw honey
½ cup white chocolate chips
2 servings CSE S'mores Protein Powder

1. Pour the cereal, graham cracker crumbs and chocolate chips into a large bowl; set aside.

2. Add the butter to a small saucepan over low heat. Once melted, add the nut butter, honey and white chocolate chips. Stir constantly until completely melted. Remove from heat and let cool for a couple minutes. Stir in one serving of the protein powder.

3. Pour the hot mixture over the top of the dry mixture in the bowl. Stir until well coated. Sprinkle with an additional serving of protein powder. Stir and serve!

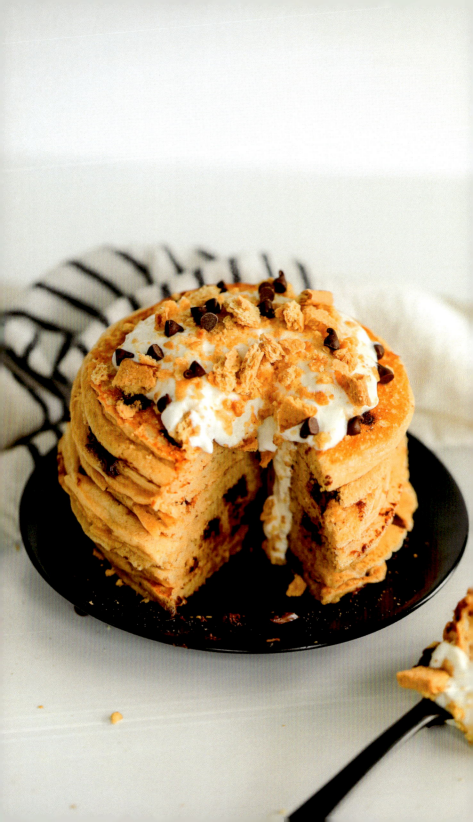

S'MORES PANCAKES

Makes 4 servings
335 calories / 7F / 37.5C / 30.5P per serving

1 ½ cups CSE Pancake & Waffle Mix
1 serving CSE S'mores Protein Powder
1 cup water
2 large eggs
Toppings per serving:
15g (about 30) chocolate chips
¼ cup nonfat, plain Greek yogurt
Vanilla stevia drops
¼ sheet of graham crackers, crumbled

1. Heat a griddle over medium heat.

2. Add all of the ingredients to a bowl and whisk together until well combined. Using a ¼ measuring cup, scoop the batter onto the greased griddle. Top each pancake with about 15 chocolate chips. Once the pancakes start to bubble on the top, flip and cook on the other side. Repeat with the remaining batter.

3. Divide the pancakes by four to get the amount to fill one serving. Should make about two pancakes per serving. Add the Greek yogurt to a bowl and stir in the stevia to sweeten. Top each serving of pancakes with ¼ cup of the sweetened yogurt and graham cracker crumbs. Enjoy!

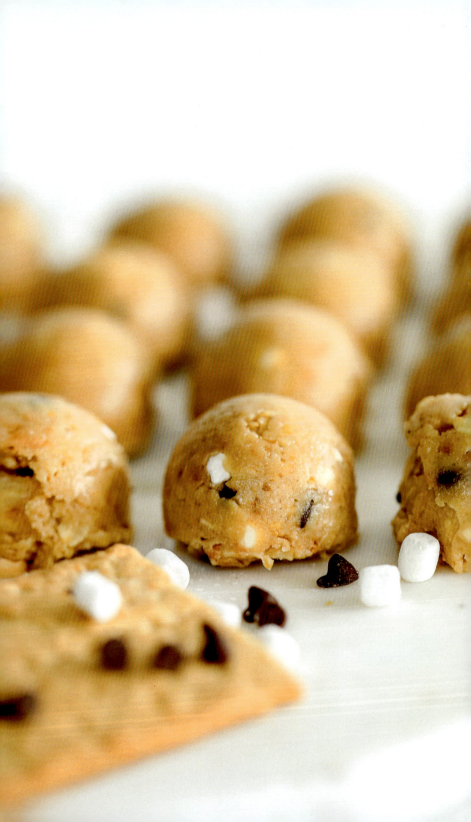

PEANUT BUTTER S'MORES POWER BITES

Makes 28 servings
105 calories / 5F / 12C / 3.5P / per ball

1 cup OffBeat Sweet Classic Peanut Butter
   or natural peanut butter
½ cup raw honey
1 serving S'mores CSE Protein Powder
1 ¼ cup old-fashioned rolled oats
2 sheet graham crackers, crumbled
2 Tbs. dried mini marshmallows
2 Tbs. mini chocolate chips
Dash sea salt

1. Add all of the ingredients to a large mixing bowl. Stir until well combined.

2. Using a small cookie scoop, scoop into balls and store them in a container in the fridge or freezer. Enjoy!

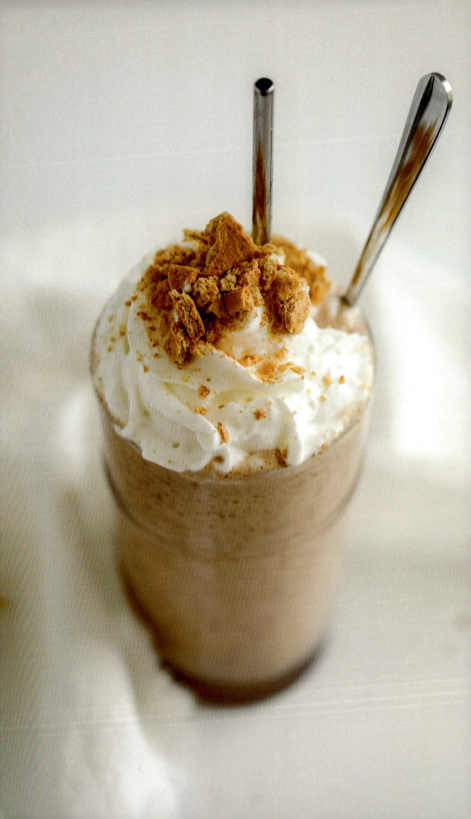

GIMME S'MORE SHAKE

Makes 1 serving
340 calories / 12F / 32C / 25P

---

1 cup unsweetened almond milk
1 serving CSE S'mores Protein Powder
½ Tbs. natural almond butter
80g frozen banana slices
10g dark chocolate chips
6-8 (120g) ice cubes
Toppings:
2 Tbs. spray whipped cream
¼ sheet of graham crackers, crumbled

1. Add all of the ingredients to a blender and blend until smooth.

2. Pour into a cup and top with the whipped cream and graham cracker crumbs. Enjoy!

SIMPLY VANILLA

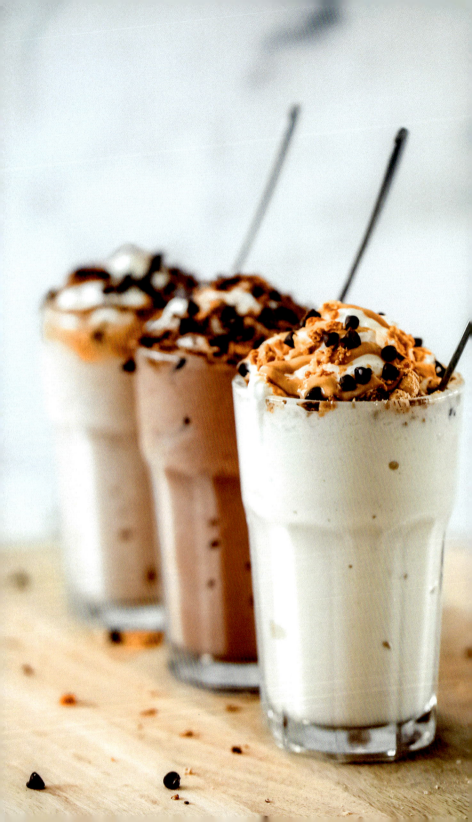

CHUNKY MONKEY MIX-IN MILKSHAKE
Makes 1 serving
400 calories / 16F / 35C / 28P

Base:
1 cup unsweetened cashew milk
1 serving CSE Simply Vanilla Protein Powder
¼ tsp. xanthan gum
150-160g ice cubes
Mix-ins:
25g Purely Elizabeth Chocolate Sea Salt + Peanut Butter
   or Banana Nut granola
12g powdered peanut butter
10g OffBeat Sweet Classic Peanut Butter, Monkey Business Butter
   or natural peanut butter
10g spray whipped cream
5g Enjoy Life mini chocolate chips

CINNAMON VANILLA MIX-IN MILKSHAKE
Makes 1 serving
355 calories / 15F / 32.5C / 25P

Base:
1 cup unsweetened cashew milk
1 serving CSE Simply Vanilla Protein Powder
¼ tsp. xanthan gum
150-160g ice cubes
Mix-ins:
25g Purely Elizabeth Original or Pumpkin Cinnamon granola
10g OffBeat Cinnamon Bun Butter or natural almond butter
10g spray whipped cream
5g Enjoy Life mini chocolate chips

1. Add all of the base ingredients to a high-powered blender.
Blend on high until smooth.

2. Pour into a cup, top with mix-ins and enjoy with a spoon!

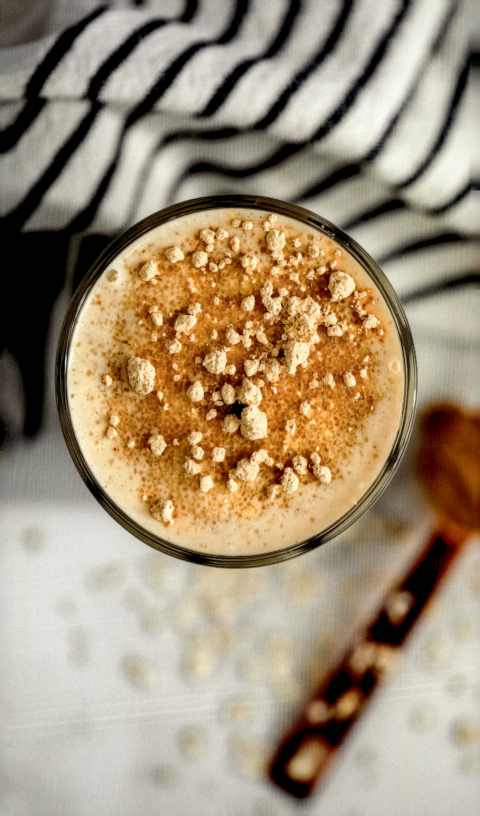

PEANUT BUTTER COOKIE BREAKFAST SHAKE

Makes 1 serving
335 calories / 9F / 33.5C / 30P

---

1 cup unsweetened almond milk
1 serving CSE Simply Vanilla Protein Powder
2 Tbs. old-fashioned rolled oats
40g frozen banana slices
2 Tbs. powdered peanut butter
1 Tbs. OffBeat Sweet Classic Peanut Butter
  or natural peanut butter
Dash sea salt
6-8 (120g) ice cubes

Topping:
1 tsp. sugar in the raw

1. Add all of the ingredients to a high-powered blender. Blend on high until smooth.

2. Sprinkle sugar in the raw on top. Enjoy!

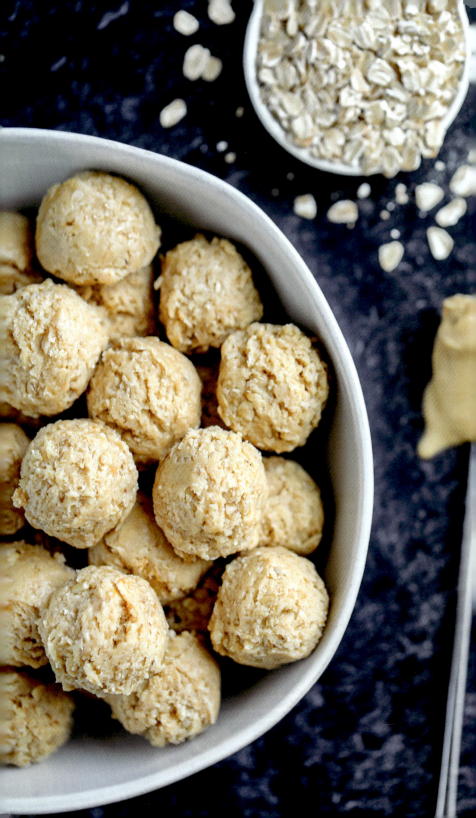

PEANUT BUTTER POWER BITES

Makes 26 bites
100 calories / 5F / 10C / 4P / per bite

1 cup OffBeat Sweet Classic Peanut Butter or natural peanut butter
½ cup raw honey
2 servings CSE Simply Vanilla Protein Powder
1 ½ cups old-fashioned rolled oats
Dash vanilla extract
Dash sea salt

(Easily prepared in a Kitchen Aid mixer)

1. Place all ingredients into a mixing bowl and stir together until well combined.

2. Scoop into balls using a small cookie scoop. Place in a conatiner and store in the fridge or freezer. Enjoy!

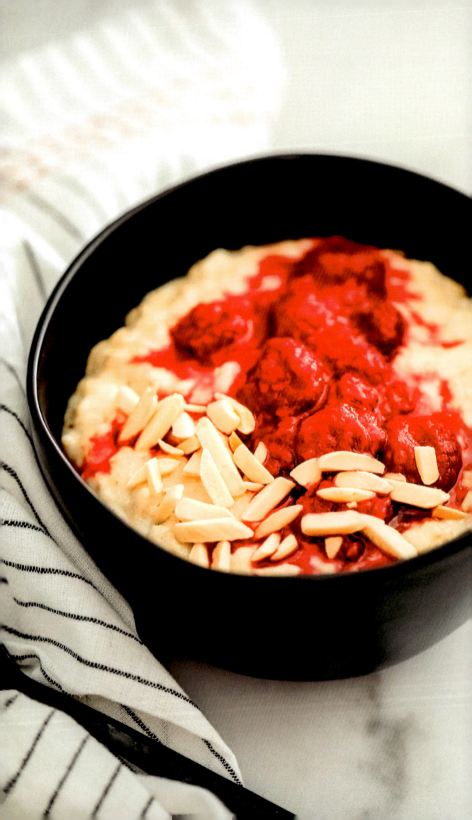

RASPBERRY ALMOND OATS

Makes 1 serving
340 calories / 10.5F / 35C / 26.5P

⅓ cup old-fashioned rolled oats
½ cup water
2 Tbs. liquid egg whites
½ Tbs. OffBeat Salted Caramel Butter or natural almond butter
⅛ tsp. almond extract
Vanilla stevia drops, optional
¼ cup nonfat, plain Greek yogurt
½ serving (17g) CSE Simply Vanilla Protein Powder
⅓ cup fresh or frozen raspberries
1 Tbs. sliced almonds

1. Mix oats, egg whites and water together in a bowl.

2. Microwave for 1-2 minutes or cook in a small pot on the stove top over medium heat for 5 minutes.

3. Stir in the nut butter of choice, almond extract, stevia and Greek yogurt. Add in the protein powder last and mix until well combined.

4. Top with raspberries and sliced almonds.

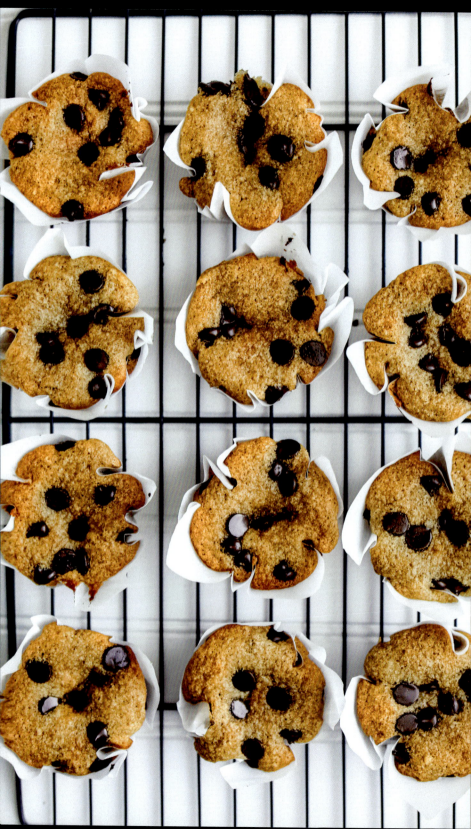

BANANA CHOCOLATE CHIP MUFFINS

Makes 13 muffins
180 calories / 6.5F / 26C / 6.5P / per muffin

2 (240g) ripe bananas
½ cup raw honey
3 Tbs. melted coconut oil
½ cup unsweetened applesauce
1 large egg
1 tsp. vanilla extract
1 ½ cups CSE Vanilla Pancake & Waffle Mix
1 serving CSE Simply Vanilla Protein Powder
2 Tbs. flaxseed meal
1 tsp. baking soda
1 tsp. baking powder
¼ tsp. sea salt

Topping per muffin:
10 dark chocolate chips (5 grams per muffin)

1. Preheat the oven to 350 degrees.

2. Mash the bananas in a large mixing bowl. Beat in the honey and coconut oil. Add in the applesauce, egg and vanilla; mix well and set aside.

3. In a separate bowl, combine the CSE Pancake & Waffle Mix, protein powder, flaxseed meal, baking soda, baking powder and sea salt. Add the wet ingredients to the dry ingredients and whisk together until just combined.

4. Line a muffin tin with liners. Scoop about ¼ cup of the batter into each muffin cup and top with chocolate chips. Bake for 15-16 minutes. Transfer from the pan to the cooling rack.

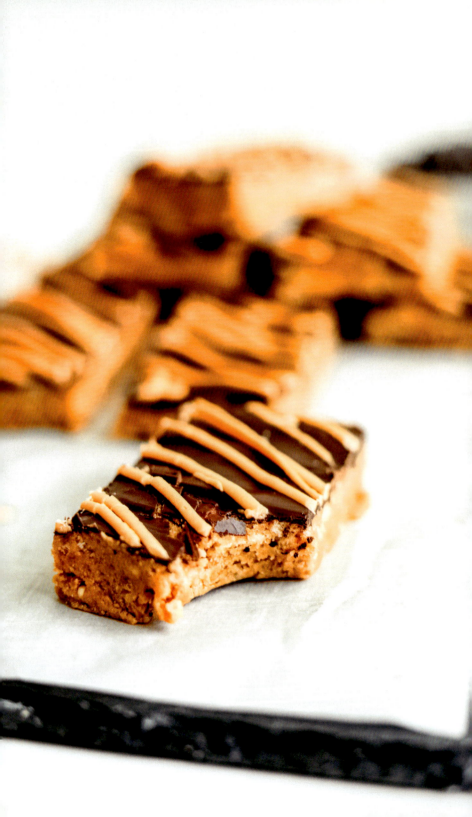

SCOTCHAROO BARS

Makes 18 bars
255 calories / 12.5F / 28.5C / 7.5P / per bar

1 cup OffBeat Sweet Classic Peanut Butter, Candy Bar Butter,
  or natural peanut butter
1 cup powdered peanut butter
¾ cup raw honey
¼ cup flaxseed meal
2 Tbs. unsweetened almond milk
1 tsp. vanilla extract
¼ tsp. sea salt
1 serving CSE Simply Vanilla Protein Powder
¼ cup butterscotch chips
2 cups Rice Krispies cereal

Toppings:
¼ cup butterscotch chips
½ cup dark chocolate chips

1. Mix the peanut butter, powdered peanut butter, honey, flaxseed meal, almond milk, vanilla extract, sea salt and protein powder together in a bowl. Melt ¼ cup of the butterscotch chips and mix in. Add the Rice Krispies cereal last and gently mix until well combined. Press into a 9x13 pan; set aside.

2. Place the chocolate chips in a bowl and microwave 30 seconds at a time until completely melted and smooth, stirring in between. Drizzle over the top of the bars and spread out smooth. Melt the remaining ¼ cup of butterscotch chips and drizzle over the top of the chocolate.

3. Store in the fridge for 1 hour to allow the chocolate to harden. Cut into 18 bars. Enjoy!

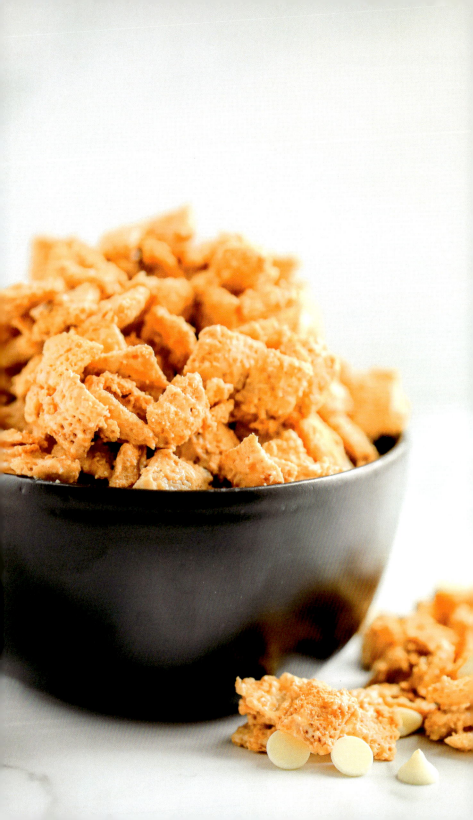

WHITE CHOCOLATE CINNAMON PUPPY CHOW

Makes 16 servings
245 calories / 11F / 29.5C / 6.5P / per serving

---

8 cups (1 box) Cinnamon Chex Cereal
2 Tbs. grass-fed butter
1 cup white chocolate chips
½ cup OffBeat Sweet Classic Peanut Butter
   or natural peanut butter
1 serving CSE Simply Vanilla Protein Powder
½ cup powdered peanut butter

1. Pour the cereal into a large bowl.

2. Add the butter, white chocolate chips and peanut butter to a small saucepan. Melt the ingredients down over low/medium heat. Whisk constantly until smooth and pourable.

3. Pour over the cereal and stir until well coated.

4. Top with the protein powder and peanut butter powder. Stir until the cereal is well coated. Weigh the entire batch and divide the weight by 16 to get the amount needed to fill one serving. Store any extras in the fridge.

SNICKERDOODLE

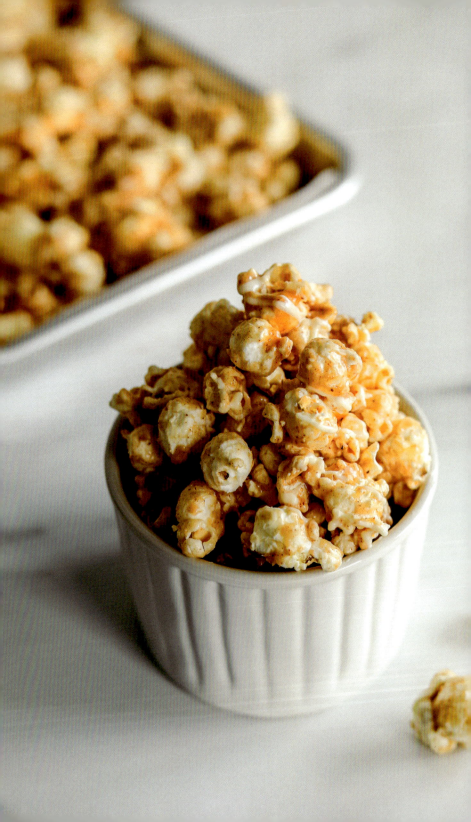

SNICKERDOODLE POPCORN

Makes 12 servings
185 calories / 5.5F / 30C / 4P / per serving

---

12 cups (½ cup kernels) air-popped popcorn
2 Tbs. white chocolate chips
¾ cup raw honey
⅓ cup OffBeat Cinnamon Bun Butter
   or natural almond butter
1 serving CSE Snickerdoodle Protein Powder
Topping:
Pinch of sea salt
¼ cup melted white chocolate chips

1. Pop the popcorn into a large bowl. Set aside.

2. Add the white chocolate chips, honey and nut butter to a saucepan over low/medium heat. Melt down together until smooth and pourable. Remove from the heat and whisk in the protein powder until smooth.

3. Pour the mixture over the popcorn and stir until the popcorn is well coated.

4. Dump out onto a baking sheet lined with parchment paper and sprinkle with sea salt.

5. Melt the chocolate chips in the microwave for 30 seconds at a time until melted and smooth, stirring in between. Usually takes 60-90 seconds total. Drizzle the white chocolate over the popcorn and allow to cool. Enjoy!

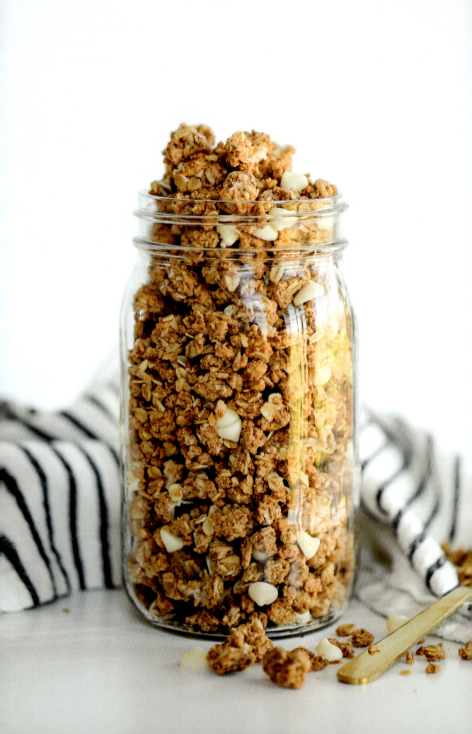

SNICKERDOODLE GRANOLA

Makes 24 servings / about 32g per serving
150 calories / 7.5F / 15C / 5P

---

12 oz. OffBeat Cinnamon Bun Butter
  or natural almond butter
½ cup raw honey
2 servings CSE Snickerdoodle Protein Powder
¼ cup flaxseed meal
2 ½ cups old-fashioned rolled oats
½ tsp. sea salt

Topping:
¼ cup white or dark chocolate chips

1. Heat the oven to 350 degrees.

2. Add the nut butter, honey, protein powder, flaxseed meal, rolled oats and salt to a mixing bowl. Stir together until well combined.

3. Dump out onto a baking sheet lined with parchment paper and spread into a single layer. Bake for 5 minutes; flip and bake another 5 minutes. Remove from oven and let cool.

4. Sprinkle with chocolate chips once cooled. Store in an airtight container in the fridge. Enjoy with milk, almond milk, on yogurt or ice cream or with a spoon.

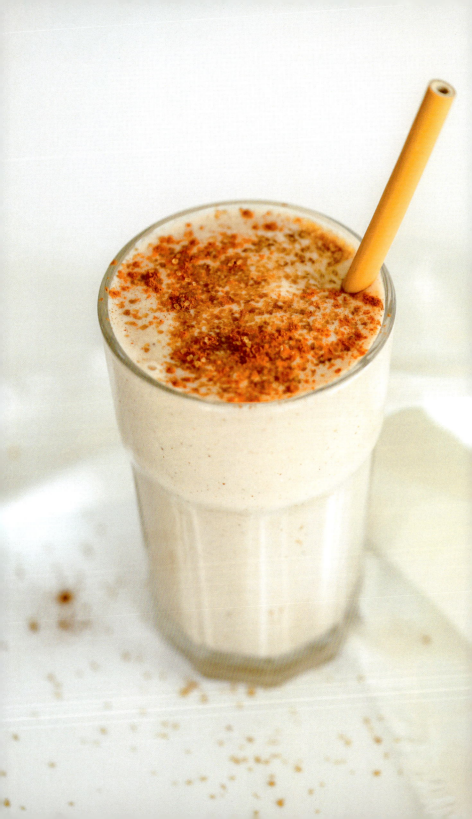

SNICKERDOODLE COOKIE SHAKE

Makes 1 serving
340 calories / 11F / 34C / 26P

1 cup unsweetened cashew milk
1 serving CSE Snickerdoodle Protein Powder
40g frozen banana slices
2 Tbs. Old-fashioned rolled oats
18g OffBeat Cinnamon Bun Butter
   or natural almond butter
6-8 (120g) ice cubes
Toppings:
Pinch of turbinado sugar
Dash of cinnamon

1. Add all of the shake ingredients to a high-powered blender. Blend on high until smooth. Pour into a cup.

2. Top with sugar and cinnamon. Enjoy!

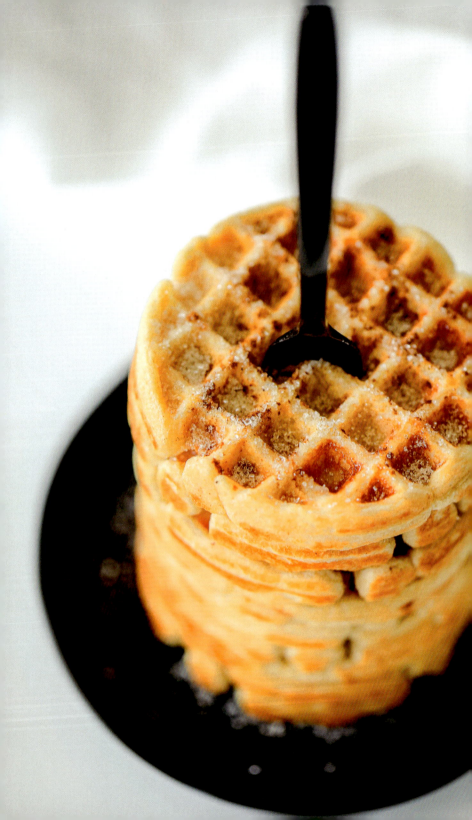

CINNAMON SUGAR WAFFLES

Makes 4 servings
270 calories / 4.5F / 33C / 25.5P per serving

2 cups CSE Vanilla Pancake & Waffle Mix
1 serving CSE Snickerdoodle Protein Powder
1 ½ cups water
2 large eggs
¼ cup nonfat, plain Greek yogurt

Toppings:
8 tsp. Sugar in the Raw
Cinnamon

1. Heat waffle iron.

2. Add the CSE Pancake & Waffle Mix, protein powder and water to a large mix-ing bowl. Mix until smooth. Whisk in the eggs and Greek yogurt.

3. Pour the batter into the hot, greased waffle iron. Once the waffle is done, keep in waffle iron, spray the top lightly with cooking spray and sprinkle with sugar and cinnamon. Close the waffle iron and cook for an additional 30 seconds. Transfer the waffle to a plate and repeat with the remainder of the batter.

4. Divide the waffles by four to get the amount needed to fill one serving. Enjoy as is or add additional toppings of choice such as your favorite yogurt, jam, berry or maple syrup (not included in the macros). Enjoy!

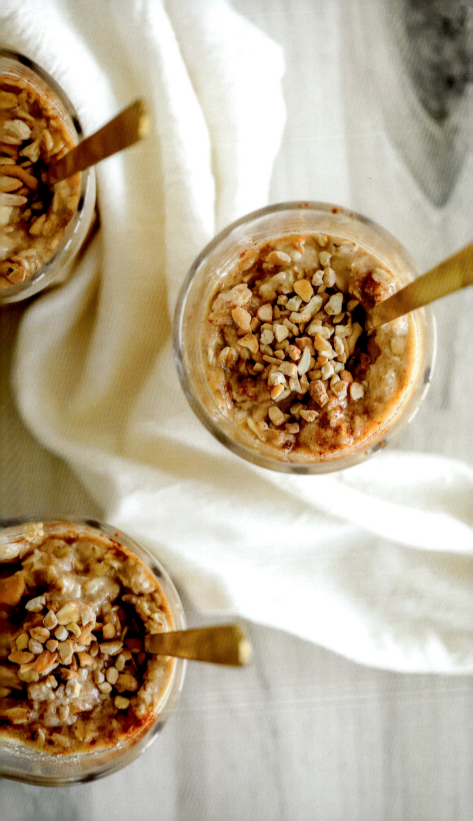

SNICKERDOODLE OVERNIGHT OATS

Makes 1 serving
365 calories / 13F / 37C / 25P

½ cup old-fashioned rolled oats
½ serving (16g) CSE Snickerdoodle Protein Powder
1 cup unsweetened vanilla almond milk
¼ cup plain, nonfat Greek yogurt
1 Tbs. (14g) OffBeat Cinnamon Bun Butter
  or natural almond butter

Toppings:
½ Tbs. chopped pecans
½ tsp. turbinado sugar
Dash of cinnamon

1. Add all the ingredients to a mason jar, cup or container. Mix until well combined.

2. Top with pecans, sugar and cinnamon. Cover and store in the fridge overnight.

3. Enjoy cold the next day. Stays good in the fridge up to 5 days.

STRAWBERRY CHEESECAKE

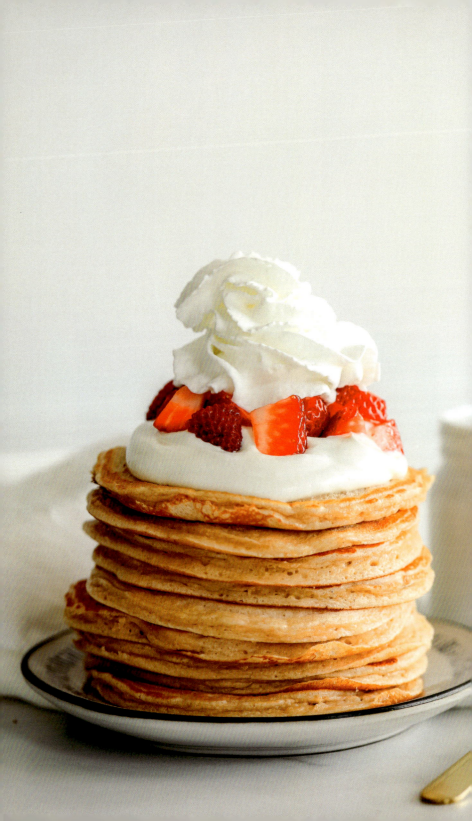

STRAWBERRIES & CREAM PANCAKES

Makes 4 servings
350 calories / 11F / 35C / 29P per serving

1 cup unsweetened vanilla almond milk
2 large eggs
1 ½ cups CSE Vanilla Pancake & Waffle Mix
2 servings CSE Strawberry Cheesecake Protein Powder
Dash sea salt
Toppings per serving:
½ Tbs. grass-fed butter
Sweetened Yogurt:
2 Tbs. nonfat, plain Greek yogurt
Vanilla stevia drops, to taste
Toppings:
½ cup fresh, chopped strawberries
2 Tbs. spray whipping cream

1. Heat griddle to medium heat.

2. Whisk the almond milk and eggs together in a large bowl. Add the CSE Pancake & Waffle Mix, Strawberry Cheesecake Protein Powder and sea salt. Whisk until well combined.

3. Using a ¼ measuring cup, pour the batter onto the greased griddle. Once small bubbles begin to form on the top, flip and cook on the other side. Divide the pancakes into four servings to get the amount needed to fill one serving.

4. In a small bowl, combine the Greek yogurt and stevia drops. Spread the butter on the pancakes, then top with the sweetened yogurt, strawberries and whipping cream.

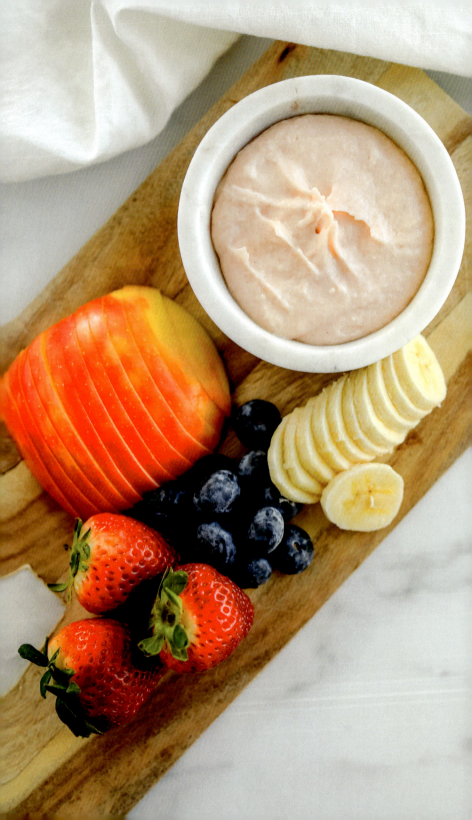

STRAWBERRY PROTEIN FRUIT DIP

Makes 1 serving
230 calories / 7F / 24C / 18P

⅓ cup nonfat, plain Greek yogurt
½ serving (16g) CSE Strawberry Cheesecake Protein Powder
1 Tbs. (14g) OffBeat Lemon Coconut Bliss Butter or
   Neufchatel cream cheese
½ Tbs. raw honey
Choose a fruit for dipping:
50g apple slices
110g strawberries
30g bananas
100g grapes

1. Add the yogurt, protein powder, OffBeat butter or cream cheese and honey to a bowl. Whisk together until smooth.

2. Use as a dip for the fruit of your choosing.

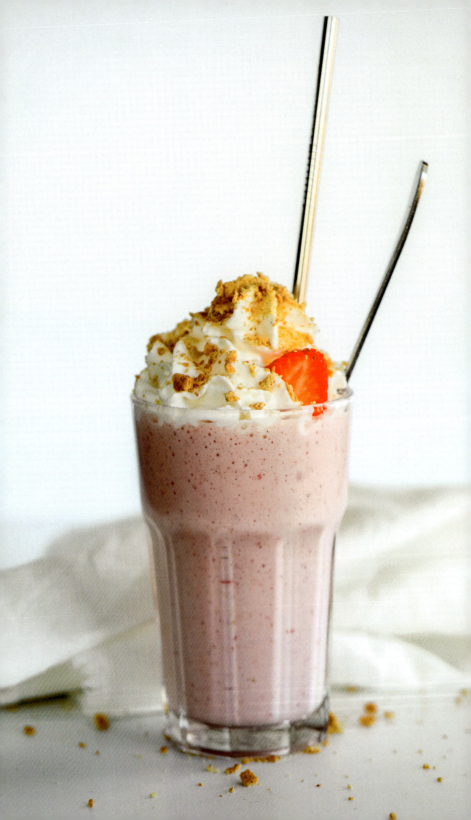

STRAWBERRY CHEESECAKE SHAKE
Makes 1 serving
330 calories / 8F / 21.5C / 18P

_____

1 cup unsweetened vanilla almond milk
½ serving (16g) CSE Strawberry Cheesecake Protein Powder
¼ cup 4% cottage cheese
100g frozen strawberries
6-8 (120g) ice cubes
Toppings:
½ sheet graham cracker, crumbled
4 Tbs. spray whipping cream

1. Add all of the shake ingredients into a high-powered blender. Blend on high until smooth. Pour into cup.

2. Top with graham cracker crumbles and spray whipping cream. Enjoy!

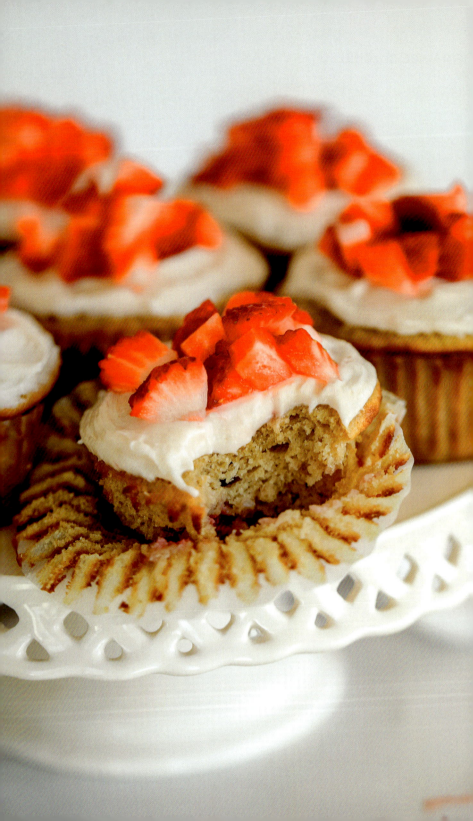

STRAWBERRY CREAM CHEESE CUPCAKES

Makes 12 cupcakes / 1 per serving
160 calories / 7F / 16.5C / 7.5P per cupcake

Cupcake Mix:
1 ½ cups CSE Vanilla Pancake & Waffle Mix
1 serving CSE Strawberry Cheesecake Protein Powder
½ cup xylitol
½ tsp. sea salt
2 tsp. baking powder
½ tsp. baking soda
1 large egg
⅓ cup unsweetened applesauce
½ cup unsweetened vanilla almond milk
2 Tbs. melted coconut oil

Cream Cheese Frosting:
4 oz. Neufchatel cream cheese
2 Tbs. grass-fed butter
¼ cup raw honey
½ tsp. vanilla extract
2 Tbs. CSE Strawberry Cheesecake Protein Powder

Topping:
1 cup sliced strawberries

1. Heat the oven to 400 degrees.

2. Make the cupcake mix by adding the CSE Pancake & Waffle Mix, protein powder, xylitol, sea salt, baking powder and baking soda to a mixing bowl. Stir until combined.

3. In a separate bowl beat the egg, applesauce, almond milk and melted coconut oil. Add the wet ingredients to the dry and mix until just combined.

4. Add muffin liners to a muffin pan. Spoon the batter into the liners using ¼ measuring cup, filling each one ¾ full. Bake for 8-10 minutes or until golden and cooked through. Transfer to a cooling rack and let cool completely before frosting.

5. Make the cream cheese frosting. Add the cream cheese to a mixing bowl and beat with hand mixers until smooth. Add the softened butter, honey and vanilla. Beat until well combined and smooth. Frost the cooled muffins and top with sliced strawberries.

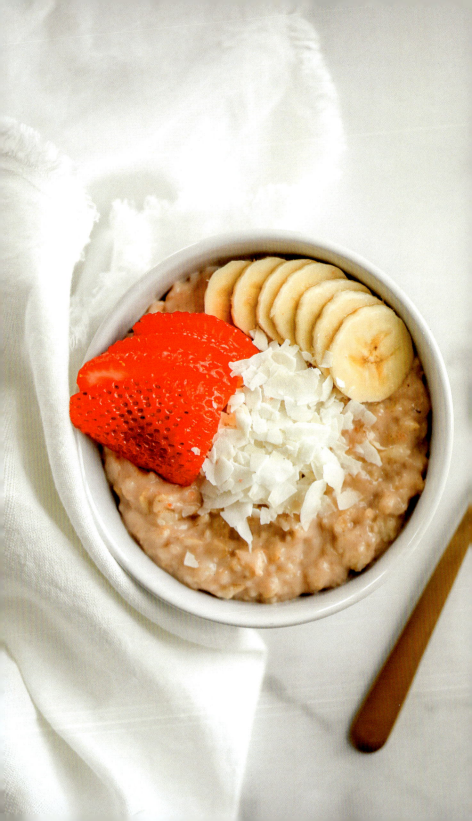

ISLAND STRAWBERRY OATMEAL

Makes 1 serving
360 calories / 12F / 37C / 25.5P

⅓ cup old-fashioned rolled oats
½ cup water
3 Tbs. (46g) liquid egg whites
1 Tbs. (14g) OffBeat Aloha Butter
   or natural almond butter
¾ serving (24g) CSE Strawberry Cheesecake Protein Powder
20g chopped banana
20g fresh, chopped strawberries
5g unsweetened shredded coconut

1. Add the oats, water and egg whites to a bowl and microwave for 1.5 minutes or cook on the stovetop over medium heat for 3-5 minutes.

2. Stir in the nut butter and let cool for 1-2 minutes. Stir in the protein powder until well combined.

3. Top with bananas, strawberries and coconut.

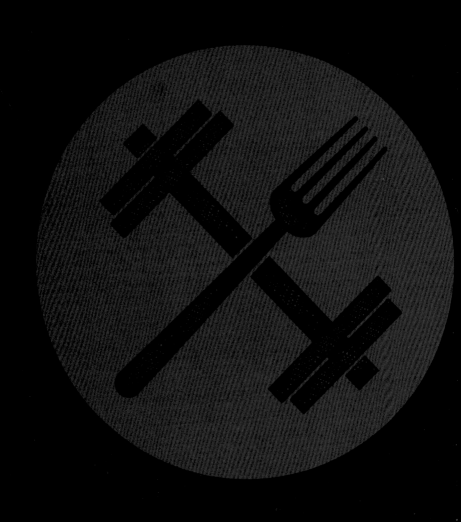

WWW.CLEANSIMPLEEATS.COM